# Retinal Detachment

THIRD EDITION

# Retinal Detachment

## THE ESSENTIALS OF MANAGEMENT

THIRD EDITION

**Hector Bryson Chawla** MB ChB (St And) DO (Lond) DRCOG (Lond) FRC (Ophth) FRCS (Ed)
Consultant Ophthalmic Surgeon Royal Infirmary, Edinburgh
Examiner, Royal College of Surgeons of Edinburgh, and Royal College of Ophthalmologists, UK
Former Fellow in the Retinal Service, North Western University, Chicago, USA
Member of the Club Jules Gonin

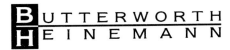

BUTTERWORTH
HEINEMANN

OXFORD  BOSTON  JOHANNESBURG  MELBOURNE  NEW DELHI  SINGAPORE

Butterworth-Heinemann
Linacre House, Jordan Hill, Oxford OX2 8DP
225 Wildwood Avenue, Woburn, MA 01801–2041
A division of Reed Educational and Professional Publishing Ltd

A member of the Reed Elsevier plc group

First published 1998

**British Library Cataloguing in Publication Data**
A catalogue record for this book is available from the British Library

**Library of Congress Cataloguing in Publication Data**
A catalogue record for this book is available from the Library of Congress

ISBN 0 7506 3980 6

Printed and bound in Great Britain
by The Bath Press plc, Avon

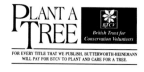

# Contents

# Foreword

I have known Dr Hector Chawla for many years, and it gives me great pleasure to provide a foreword to the latest edition of his justly admired book on retinal detachment.

The book, and its success in previous editions, are ample demonstration of Hector Chawla's mastery of this complex and important topic. What the book cannot show, however, is something that patients prize every bit as much in their doctors as technical excellence, namely those human qualities of compassion, reassurance and the ability to communicate – qualities I know the author to possess in the highest degree.

A long time ago, on a school playing field, I experienced the first symptoms of the condition that is the subject of this book. Somewhat later I met Hector Chawla. To this day I am grateful to him, and indebted to his skills.

His book is aimed at professionals, indeed at experts, and like others he has written, it enjoys high professional regard. As one who has met the author, and benefited from his expertise, I am glad to know that this expertise continues to be passed on, in this third edition, to his professional colleagues all over the world.

*Rt Hon Gordon Brown MP, Chancellor of the Exchequer*

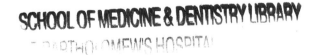

# Preface

New truths, according to Thomas Huxley, begin life as heresies and end as superstitions. Jules Gonin's demonstration that a hole in the retina would lead to a retinal detachment and that sealing this hole would lead to a cure, was certainly new and predictably greeted with disbelief. Despite its initial cool reception, his discovery remains today not a superstition but an eternal truth.

Once the need to treat a retinal break was established, the next requirement was to see it. In the English-speaking world in particular, the favoured direct ophthalmoscope generally managed a view of sorts up to the equator, leaving the rest, where it mattered, to the imagination.

Charles Schepens, the next great figure in the story, changed all that. With the binocular indirect ophthalmoscope he not only saw the retina up to the ora serrata, but he described it in some detail as well. The door was now open for famous names to contribute to the development of what is today called conventional retinal surgery, with a functional success rate previously inconceivable.

This very success, however, revealed pathological influences hitherto unconsidered because they had no relevance in the redetachment of a retina that had not yet been flattened. 'Touch not the vitreous' used to be an ophthalmic axiom until Robert Machemer not only touched it, but also removed it. Thus one of the major advances in ophthalmic surgery of this century was introduced, raising a whole range of therapeutic possibilities that would have been regarded as delusional not that long ago.

This book hopes to merge these two pathways into one broad approach to the successful surgery of disorders of the retina and the vitreous.

# About the author

Hector Chawla started the Retina Service in the Royal Infirmary, Edinburgh, UK. In the years immediately following a Retinal Fellowship in Chicago, USA, in 1968, he published extensively on the use of the intravitreal air, a technique now accepted throughout the world as beyond question.

Mr Chawla is consultant in charge of the Retinal Service in Edinburgh; he is a member of the Club Jules Gonin and examiner to the Royal Colleges of Surgeons of Edinburgh and Glasgow and the College of Ophthalmologists, UK. He is a member of the Advisory Board in Ophthalmology of the Edinburgh College and Visiting Lecturer to the M Med (Ophthalmology) course, School of Postgraduate Medical Studies, National University of Singapore, Republic of Singapore.

He has published several scientific papers, three textbooks as sole author, one as joint author, one as contributor and one novel.

# Acknowledgements

My grateful thanks are due to my secretary Mrs Sandra McDonagh, who responded to every change of mind with a smile, and to Mr Terry Tarrant, whose illustrations have all the crispness and elegance that we have come to take for granted. None of the techniques described in this text would have been possible without the help, enthusiasm and expert collaboration of our theatre nurses, led by Mrs Jackie MacDonald.

My special thanks are due to my colleague Dr Jaswinder Singh, recently a Fellow of the Lions Institute in Perth, Western Australia, for his advice and help in the planning of the chapter on vitrectomy and for scanning the manuscript for undetected flaws.

My special thanks will always be due to the late Dr J. Graham Dobbie, of North Western University, Chicago, whose surgical skill remains in my memory as magical as it was when I first worked with him.

# 1

# The binocular indirect ophthalmoscope

The binocular indirect ophthalmoscope is the linchpin of successful retinal surgery, yet it has a reputation for complexity, providing a fleeting, elusive and, worse, an inverted image. This gives the direct ophthalmoscope, by contrast, a spurious charm.

**Figure 1.1**
Parallel rays of light from the fundus are brought to an inverted focus on the observer's side of the viewing lens.

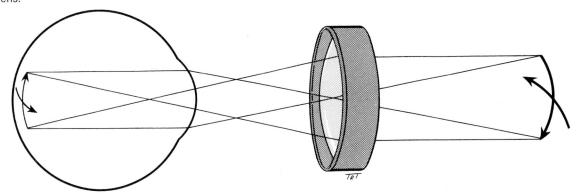

Such a reputation is totally unjustified and just one of the following advantages should be enough in its own right to claim pride of place for the binocular indirect ophthalmoscope. Taken together, they make the claim irrefutable.

The indirect ophthalmoscope has five main advantages.
1. The beam can penetrate most medial opacities
2. The reduced image allows an overall assessment of the retina at a glance
3. The refractive error of the patient is irrelevant
4. The binocular sense of depth allows the surgeon to relate the positions of the intraocular contents to one another in three dimensions
5. The possibility of surgical contamination is greatly reduced.

The secret of mastery is the old military standby of divide and rule – to break the unbreakable into its elements and to pick them off one by one.

# THE HEAD PIECE

The headband can be adjusted to fit heads of all shapes and sizes, but having a personal lamp obviates the need for recurrent irritating re-adjustment. Once the instrument is placed on the head, the distance between the eye pieces may require alteration in order to let the observer achieve a binocular focus on the illuminated fingertips of the extended hand at arms length.

**Figure 1.2**
Movement in an anteroposterior direction allows the casing to bring the viewing holes close to the eye. Sideways movement of these viewing holes accommodates the interpupillary distance of most observers.

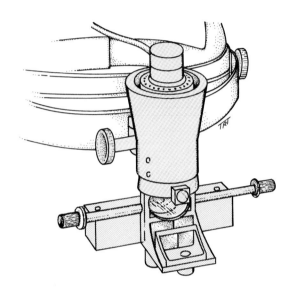

**Figure 1.3**
The beam captures the fingertips of the outstretched hand.

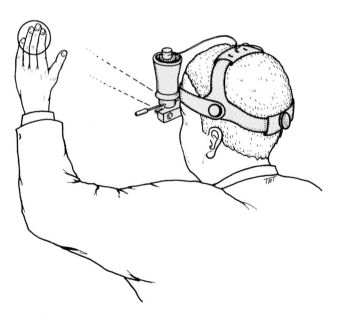

Positioning the eye pieces as close to the face as comfort will allow removes most of the difficulties, and recent instrument design has simplified things still further.

**Figure 1.4**
The standard position for fundal examination. Viewing from 5cm (focal distance 20 D lens) creates a useful microscope in the operating room.

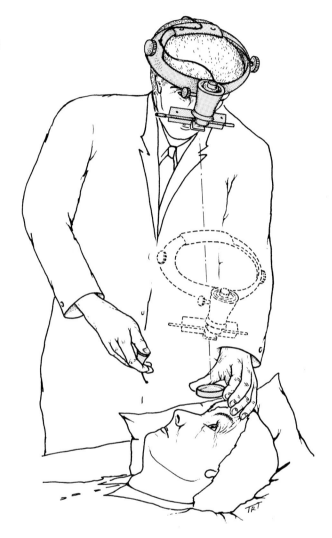

Although not all clinic rooms boast an examination couch, the instrument clearly comes into its own with the patient recumbent. Most areas within the fundus are easily accessible, but the lower retina tends to be lost in shimmering reflexes when the examiner gazes directly down into the lower quadrants. A slight turn towards the left side (if the lens is held in the left hand) or to the right (if the lens is held in the right hand) lights up the inferior quadrants with an oblique beam, and replaces the shimmer with fundal detail.

It must be remembered that the light is painfully fierce. A patient is much more likely to cooperate with a dipped beam, or even better, with a tinted 20 dioptre lens.

## THE LENS

The inverted retinal image hangs in space before a powerful convex lens, and it is the difficulty encountered in holding this image that may persuade people to stay with a more familiar constant direct view.

The correct way to hold the lens is between the thumb and forefinger of the left or right hand, with the more curved surface away from the patient. Although the lens should be kept as nearly parallel to the iris plane as possible, it must be tilted slightly to avoid a 90° angle to the main beam. Each lens surface reflects this beam like a mirror, and tilting the lens slightly separates the two reflections that would otherwise conceal the inner eye with a flood of light.

There are several types of lenses to suit all tastes, but different combinations of surface and curvature claim different qualities and a yellow-tinted lens is unquestionably kinder to the patient. The most popular strength is +20 dioptres, combining the advantage of the overall field size with sufficient magnification to give some purpose to the examination. Lenses of +15 dioptres give images of increased size, but their increased focal distance is a torture to short fingers. Furthermore, the larger image is still more elusive, and this seems to defeat the whole point of the wide viewing field. However, this must be a matter of choice and of finger length.

Whichever lens is chosen, its surfaces must be treated with reverence. A few scratches or thumb prints will obscure what a cloudy vitreous will not. Holding the lens in the non-dominant hand liberates the master hand to wield the scleral depressor, the cotton tipped applicator or the cryoprobe. The temptation to apply the dominant hand to the lens is strong, but should be resisted.

Some surgeons do hold the lens in the master hand, manipulating the probes very skilfully with the weaker hand. It is possible, however, that so doing makes the search for mastery somewhat longer.

Most people travel this far, and then give up after the first futile attempts to secure a retinal picture. Why they do so is perfectly understandable. Their concentration is divided between what is seen and where it is seen, and their thoughts are split between what they hope they see, what they think they see, where it came from if the surgeon or the patient moved, and where it will go should either move again.

It is easier to learn the technique if it is studied in two parts; first learn how to hold the image without effort, and then learn about its possible movements. Trying to do both things at the same time can only lead to failure.

## THE INVERTED IMAGE

In order to hold a continuous retinal view, the procedure should always be carried out with the patient lying down. The upright position exhausts the patient's neck, the examiner's lens arm and the tolerance of both.

Once the image can be held as long as the surgeon chooses and is not at the mercy of a flood of tears and orbicularis spasm, the next step is to turn that fleeting visual impression into a permanent record. Just as not holing out every putt may flatter a golf score, so not drawing the fundus may create the illusion that indirect ophthalmology has been mastered.

Drawing the fundus exposes any gaps in the imagined quality of understanding. The fundi being drawn need not be unhealthy, and dipping the examining beam will ensure that they stay that way.

Although the interior of the eye curves forwards like a brandy glass with the diameter of the ora narrower than that of the equator, creating and storing a record in this form would clearly be impossible. Convention reduces the detachment chart to a flat circle, with the outer contour line representing the ora serrata and the inner one the equator. The chart should be placed upside down on the patient's chest and the visualized images recorded as they appear. The examiner does not of course stand in one place, but moves freely from one side to the other all the way round the patient's head – manoeuvres that are duplicated in the operating room.

**Figure 1.5**
A retinal detachment with an upper temporal horseshoe tear in the right eye of a myope as recorded during binocular ophthalmoscopy.

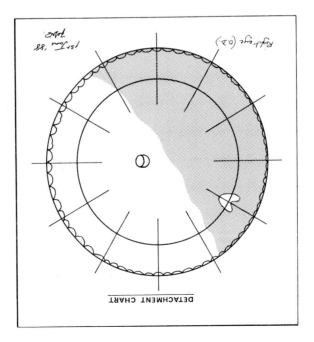

The arterioles and venules twine and branch and taper towards the pigment-stippled ora, and a degree of accuracy is required if their position in the eye is to be transferred precisely to paper. Ten such drawings will rapidly bring a degree of fluency that we might never have dared to expect initially.

The inverted image must be accepted as a natural state of affairs and not just as an optical anomaly. The inversion is total, with not only the meridian but also points on the meridians – connecting as contour lines parallel to the limbus and the ora serrata – reversed.

The vortex ampullae on the equator of the eye are in similar positions, but differ in appearance. Each bears a loose resemblance to an octopus, with a body and an apparent superfluity of legs. This happy variation can be used to illustrate how features seen in the eye are reversed in three dimensions in the condensing lens. For example, the equator of the retina at 12 o'clock identified by a vortex ampulla will be seen at 6 o'clock in the lens, the 1 o'clock meridian – the fork tail of the ampulla – comes into view at 7 o'clock in the lens, and the 11 o'clock meridian – the rounded knuckle of the ampulla – must then be seen at 5 o'clock in the lens.

**Figure 1.6**
Everything is inverted – the meridians around the clock face and the contour lines that connect these meridians in three dimensions from the disc to the ora serrata.

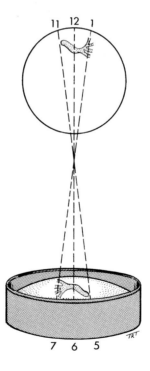

It must not be forgotten that the anterior and posterior margins are also reversed. If we think of them as contour lines on a map, the concave anterior edge presenting up towards the ora serrata between 11 and 1 o'clock will appear in the lens down towards the ora serrata between 5 and 7 o'clock, and the convex posterior edge presenting down towards the posterior pole between 11 and 1 o'clock will appear in the lens up towards the posterior pole between 5 and 7 o'clock.

Everything is reversed, and remembering this must become a habit.

## THE EFFECT OF MOVEMENTS

The following three rules of movement, like multiplication tables and grammar, if driven into the subconscious brain will not be forgotten when they are most needed The effort required to learn them by heart is considerably less than that required to recall them when they are half-learned and half-forgotten, and this effort becomes even less when we realize that all three movements are variations on a single theme – a rondo on the posterior segment of the eye.

1. The examiner can change the viewing point by moving over the concave surface of the retina
2. The examiner can move an object over the convex surface of the sclera – a cotton bud, a scleral depressor or a cryo-probe

**Figure 1.7**
The first 'against' movement. The lens and observer move in one direction and the image perceived in the lens moves in the opposite direction.

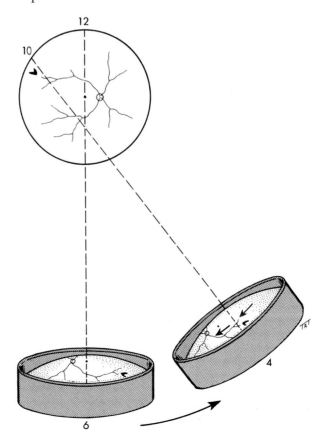

3. When the eye is described as moving in any direction, the description in fact refers to movements of the cornea – the front wall of the eye. The posterior wall of the eye, of course, rotates in the opposite direction.

**Figure 1.8**
The second 'against' movement. A scleral depressor or its equivalent moves in one direction and the image perceived in the lens moves in the opposite direction.

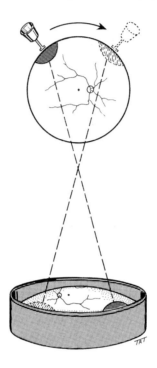

**Figure 1.9**
The apparent 'with' movement. The anterior pole of the eye moves in one direction, and the image of the posterior pole perceived in the lens moves in the same direction.

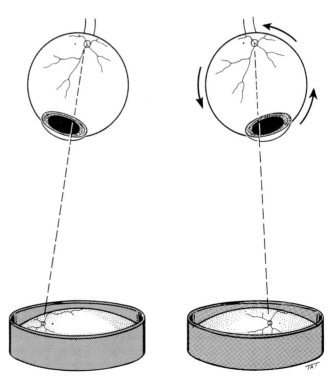

With the first two movements, the perceived image in the lens moves in the opposite direction – an 'against' movement. With the third movement, the perceived image in the lens moves in the same direction as the cornea – a 'with' movement. This is really an 'against movement' in relation to the posterior pole, but clearly no-one asks a patient to turn the optic nerves to the left when they want the eyes to turn to the right.

These movements take place of course not just from meridian to meridian around the clock face, but also from contour line to contour line from the disc to the ora serrata.

## REFERENCES AND FURTHER READING

Giraud-Teulon, M. A. L. F. (1861). Ophthalmoscopie binoculaire. *Ann. Id'oc.*, **45**, 232–250.

Schepens, C. L. (1947). A new ophthalmoscope demonstration. *Transact. Amer. Acad. Ophthalmol.: Autolaryngol.*, **51**, 298.

# 2

# Scleral depression

The technique of scleral depression is a critical element in retinal surgery for two reasons. First, it permits a dynamic inspection of that area of the retina between the equator and the ora serrata far beyond the limits of the direct ophthalmoscope, where so much significant retinal pathology may be found. Rolling the peripheral retina over the hump of the scleral depressor throws the retinal surface into relief against little hillocks and hollows, and so displays features which are visible but not identifiable without indentation. Secondly, the same technique of depression forms the foundation for the necessary and accurate placing of the cryoprobe and the location of retinal breaks during surgery.

The classic scleral depressor is rather like a thimble with a curving rim and a crossbar, and was originally intended to be worn on the fingertip. However, retinal surgeons wield it rather differently, with the thumb occluding the opening and the stem under the control of the index and middle fingers.

**Figure 2.1**
The scleral depressor.

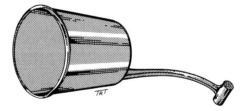

Most of the retinal periphery can be reached with scleral depression through the eyelids, but that on the 9 and 3 o'clock meridians may be elusive to begin with. Rather than bruise the lids and the patient's confidence, direct application of the crossbar to the eyeball after topical anaesthesia is quite in order. As facility develops, however, the vital contour lines at the nasal end of the horizontal meridian from the equator to the ora serrata can also be detected through the lids. The secret is to turn the patient's eye back from the absolute extremes of gaze towards the primary position. If the ophthalmoscopic beam is to maintain its connection with the eye it has to move in the same direction, and since the ophthalmoscope

**Figure 2.2**
The depressor in action. The tip is insinuated in the fold of the upper eyelid with the eye pointing in a direction opposite to that of the desired examination. The shaft must be as near parallel to the scleral surface as possible.

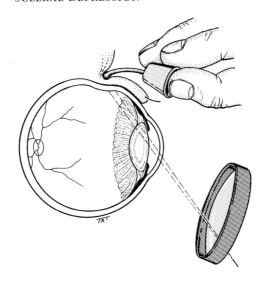

**Figure 2.3**
The correct way to position the depressor.

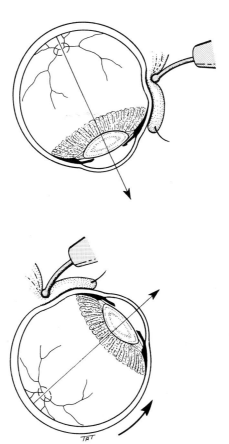

**Figure 2.4**
A paperclip makes an excellent substitute for the real thing.

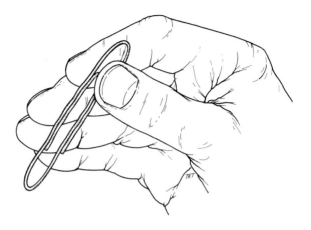

**Figure 2.5**
The easiest way to visualize the indented nasal ora serrata on the horizontal meridian – the eye pointing almost to the ceiling and the examining beam nearing the horizontal.

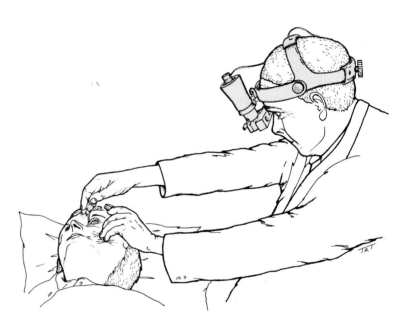

is strapped to the examiner's head, that too must move. If the patient is recumbent, this means that the examiner's line of gaze shifts away from the vertical towards the horizontal. The same result can be achieved by half turning the patient's head whilst keeping the eyes in the primary position in relation to the new position of the head.

As with all art forms technique is not everything, but without technique there is nothing. The art is to warn the patient of the pressure on the eyelid before attempting to place the crossbar beyond the tarsal plate, with the eye turned away from the intended direction of study. As the eye then rotates into the study position, it carries the depressor into the soft fold of the eyelid and raises a mobile mound, visible through the examining lens. This mobility allows lesions to be assessed in three dimensions with changing shape and profile.

**Figure 2.6**
The lens hand should lean on the
cheek and the indenting hand on the
forehead – if this is painful, it is being
done incorrectly.

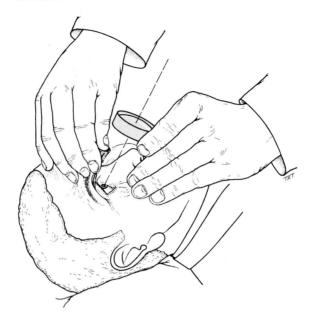

**Figure 2.6**
The lens hand should lean on the cheek and the indenting hand on the forehead – if this is painful, it is being done incorrectly.

Movement of the depressor in one direction produces a movement of the indenting image in the lens in the opposite direction. This parallels exactly the 'against' movements seen in the lens when the examiner's head moves the beam. Movement backward and forwards to pick up the anteroposterior contour lines follows the same rule, and flattening the stem of the depressor towards the eye surface with a firm but gentle pressure reveals maximal information with minimal discomfort to the patient (see Figure 1.8).

## REFERENCES AND FURTHER READING

Rosenthal, M. L. (1981). The technique of binocular indirect ophthalmoscopy. In *Retinal Detachment – A Manual Prepared for the Use of Graduates in Medicine* (G. F. Hilton, E. B. McLean, E. W. D. Norton, eds.) pp. 117–154, *Am. Acad. Ophthalmol.*

Schepens, C. L. (1969). Techniques of examination of the fundus periphery. *Trans. of the New Orleans Acad. Ophthal. Symposium on Retina and Retinal Surgery, St Louis*, pp. 39–51. Mosby, 1969.

# 3

# The pathology of retinal detachment

A retinal detachment is not really a detachment of the complete retina, but rather the separation of the neural component from the pigment component. The neural retina can be pulled off by vitreoretinal traction or raised by exudation or by a tumour, but damage most commonly occurs when a break in its surface permits aqueous or liquified vitreous to pass from the vitreal cavity into the potential space that exists between the two retinal layers. However, as long as we are aware of exactly which portion of the retina is detaching, only a pedant would seek to discard a clinical title so firmly established in ophthalmic parlance.

A break in the retinal surface alone is not enough to give rise to detachment. Fluid can only collect beneath the neuro-retina if it is both available and has access to the retinal break. Such circumstances arise when the vitreal gel collapses and separates the vitreal cortex from the retinal surface. Aetiologically, retinal breaks may result either from some induced weakness in the retina itself or from some apparent interplay between the retina and the vitreous.

**Figure 3.1**
A retina detaches because of the passage of fluid vitreous through an open break. Traction adds to the retinal separation.

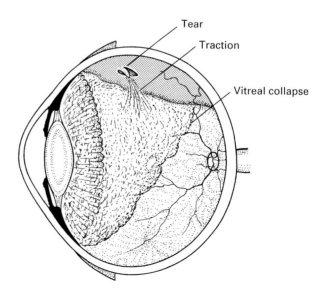

Tear

Traction

Vitreal collapse

## CONGENITAL DETACHMENT

### Dialysis

Although it may appear a simplistic explanation, the cells in the developing retina have most demands put upon them in the lower temporal quadrant of the eye. It is not surprising, therefore, that their failure to develop fully gives rise to spontaneous cracks that open and spread parallel to the ora serrata, often with small subsidiary slits at either extremity.

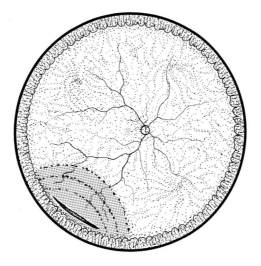

**Figure 3.2**
A lower temporal dialysis arrested on three occasions, each shown by a new 'tide mark'. The next 'high tide' will sweep the retinal detachment into the macula.

Because this is a congenital problem it tends to be found in the younger age group, where the vitreous is relatively healthy. A solid vitreous in combination with gravity militates against a fast-spreading retinal detachment. Whatever the elevation, each detachment produces irritation, which in turn causes an inflammatory reaction. The inflammatory process forms a pigmented line at the posterior edge of the retinal elevation, and this tide mark or high water mark might be regarded as an attempt by the eye to treat its own detachment. Such attempts however are usually in vain, and can be recognized by the multiplicity of curving stippled lines that may be seen following a detachment that becomes evident only when it touches the macula.

If a congenital weakness affects one eye, something sinister is frequently to be found lurking in the other.

## DEGENERATIVE DETACHMENT

A myopic eye, equally simplistically, might be considered to have a retina which is too thin in places and fails to cover a large surface area adequately. Patches of atrophy coupled with abnormal vitreal adhesion can be found scattered around the equator, where they are given the name of lattice degeneration. This is recognized by pigmentary clumps, or classically by a little crisscross in white, for all the world like trellis work.

**Figure 3.3**
Lattice degeneration and the formation of retinal breaks. There is no traction on round holes, which are frequently asymptomatic. Traction on the operculum of a horseshoe break produces flashing lights and floaters.

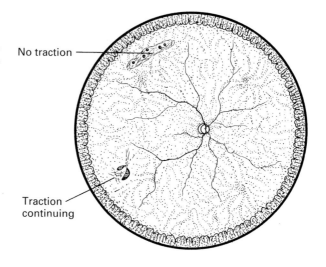

### Round holes
Simple atrophy in a patch of lattice can connect the vitreal cavity with the subretinal space.

Occasionally traction can tear a round fragment from the retina which can be seen floating in the vitreous (no longer dragging on the retina) and almost beckoning the examiner towards the retinal hole.

### Horseshoe break
Traction on an abnormal vitreoretinal adhesion can pull on the retina sufficiently to tear the adherent area away from the rest. The resultant form is typically that of a horseshoe, with the convex edge of the hoof pointing towards the disc, and the lattice change crisscrossing the operculum in the concavity dragging towards the ora serrata.

### Giant tear
This may be degenerative or congenital, but it must be assumed that, in the absence of trauma, a giant tear will develop in an eye that has a degree of malformation affecting both the retina and the vitreous, threatening 360° of the retina between the equator and the ora serrata. Abnormal adhesion of the vitreous to the posterior or anterior layers can, of course, affect the surgical outcome. Since a gap parallel to the ora serrata exists between the anterior and posterior frills

of the retina, it might be reasonable to regard a giant tear as an extended dialysis, but with the posterior lip dragged by vitreal adhesion towards the disc

To merit the title 'giant', the rent has to extend over at least 90° of the retinal periphery.

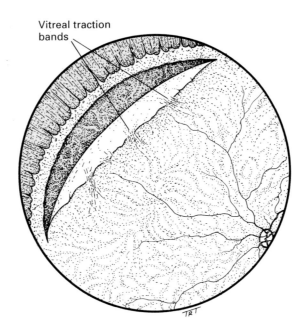

Vitreal traction bands

**Figure 3.4**
A giant tear – a dialysis with vitreous attached to the posterior lip and a peripheral frill of intact retina.

## TRAUMATIC DETACHMENT

Injury can take many forms, and perhaps the commonest is surgery of one kind or another.

### Aphakia
Cataract extraction, particularly by the intracapsular method, allows the vitreous to move forward into the space originally occupied by the lens. Since the vitreous base straddles the ora, such forward movement allows a degree of traction on the peripheral retina at the posterior limit of the vitreous base where it can produce tiny, and often multiple, horseshoe breaks. Extracapsular extraction complicated by vitreous loss creates the same tiny multiple breaks.

The presence of pseudophakia does not necessarily mean that tears are aphakic. The patient may be a myope whose cataract extraction has triggered a myopic retinal detachment.

### Yag capsulotomy
The constant desire for perfection – to turn 6/12 into 6/5 vision – can sometimes create the reverse, and cause lack of

perception of light. The act of penetrating the capsule sends shockwaves through the vitreal cavity, and the very existence of the new opening may create the same circumstances as in intracapsular cataract extraction. Together, these events can awaken catastrophic activity in existing vitreoretinal pathology that might have continued to slumber happily behind a slightly thickened but intact capsule.

**Figure 3.5**
Classic aphakic tears at the posterior edge of the vitreous base; the result of forward movement of the vitreous dragging on the vitreoretinal demarcation line.

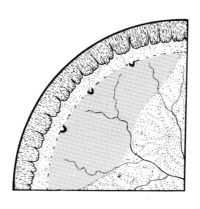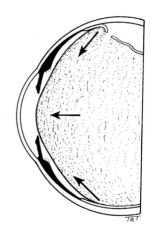

### Strabismus surgery

The custom of allowing embryo surgeons to cut their surgical teeth on squints has little to be said in its favour. A needle intended for the sclera only may slide into the cavity of the eye, involving all the layers both on entry and again on exit. Only the health of the youthful vitreous saves the surgeon from adding the visual defect of a detached retina to the existing cosmetic problem.

### Vitrectomy

The active manipulation of a probe through the pars plana just ahead of the temporal and nasal ora serrata not infrequently tears the peripheral retina. Such a possibility must be considered, watched for and treated prophylactically at the end of every vitrectomy.

### Disinsertion

Frequently but wrongly regarded as synonymous with a dialysis, a disinsertion is in fact quite different. It is a response to injury, and occurs when the ora serrata itself is torn from its moorings. Lacerated ribbons of ciliary epithelium may form the anterior border. The oral scallops hang free in the vitreal cavity and frequently in vitreal blood as well.

Although textbooks often state that the upper nasal ora is the area most at risk, in practice a disinsertion is most likely to be found in the lower temporal quadrants.

**Figure 3.6**
Manipulation of the vitreal suction cutter is a common cause of disinsertion of the upper temporal and upper nasal ora serrata. Attempts to spare the natural lens make these breaks more likely.

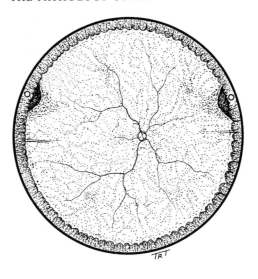

**Figure 3.7**
Disinsertion avulsion of the ora serrata and sometimes of the ciliary epithelium is brought about by trauma. The detachment may then resemble that of a dialysis, but the underlying pathology is very different.

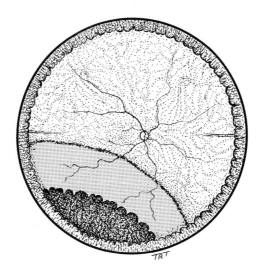

### Macular hole (traumatic)

The contre-coup waves from frontal injury can shock the macular retina which, after losing acuity, may eventually lose its integrity as a sharp-edged round hole. The shock of injury occasionally produces sufficient inflammatory glue to hold everything together, but often it does not.

### Macular hole (spontaneous)

Extreme myopia can result in a full-thickness break at the macula; in the absence of this, spontaneous macular holes may also occasionally be found postmenopausal women. No studies have been carried out to consider the possible influence of hormone replacement therapy.

**Random injury**

Trauma by its very nature is not usually directed with precision, and a breach in the retina may appear as a remote effect of blunt trauma, whereas sharp-edged trauma will lacerate wherever it strikes.

## LONG-STANDING DETACHMENT

Retinal elevations of long duration show some or all of the following features:
1. Recent macular involvement, giving the spurious impression of a recent detachment
2. Iritic adhesions and pigment clumps on the lens
3. Relative hypotony (unless the pupil is blocked)
4. Posterior subcapsular cataract
5. Grey-white curtains of organized vitreal blood
6. Round blobs of vitreal debris
7. Tide marks
8. Rigid immobile retina
9. Full thickness retinal cysts, which disappear after successful surgery.

## REFERENCES AND FURTHER READING

Dumas, J. and Schepens, C. L. (1966). Chorioretinal lesions predisposing to retinal breaks. *Am. J. Ophthalmol.*, **61**, 620–630.

Foulds, W. S. (1987). Is your vitreous really necessary? The role of the vitreous in the eye with particular reference to retinal attachment, detachment and the mode of action of vitreous substitutes. *Eye*, **1**, 641–664.

Gonin, J. (1923). Guerisons operatoires de decollements retiniens. *Rev. Gen. Ophthalmol.*, **37**, 337–340.

Machemer, R. (1984). The importance of fluid resorption, traction, intraocular currents and chorioretinal scars in therapy of rhegmatogenous retinal detachments. *Am. J. Ophthalmol.*, **98**, 681–693.

Morse, P. H. (1974). Lattice degeneration of the retina and retinal detachment. *Am. J. Ophthalmol.*, **78**, 930–934.

# 4

# Clinical features

The pathological sequence resulting in a retinal break, the creation of the break itself and the detachment of the retina (which may or may not follow the break) can cause a number of symptoms which may range from a slight disturbance of vision to total loss of light perception. The patient's complaints will vary depending on the speed of the process, the point at which the complaint is made, whether it has happened before to the other eye and, finally, on the temperament of the patient in question.

Not all flashing lights and floaters indicate a retinal detachment, but they must be taken seriously as a possible prelude to the formation of at least a retinal break. Sudden loss of vision in this context may be due to either a retinal haemorrhage, a retinal detachment, or both. Creeping loss of vision, particularly with the development of a shadow, must be taken as grave evidence that the retina is beginning to detach.

**Figure 4.1**
The classic symptoms of a retinal detachment – flashing lights, floaters and a 'black curtain' rising across the visual field. The latter may be neither black nor a curtain, but rather a sense of flickering that will not go away. The clearest indication that the retina is detaching is loss of the choroidal pattern.

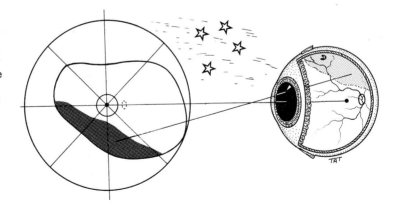

SYMPTOMS

**Flashing lights**
Retinal sensation is light-specific, and any disturbance of the retina or of the visual cortex will give rise to some sort of aberrant light awareness.

Flashes of vitreoretinal origin may signify that:
1. The vitreous is making abnormal movements
2. The retina is tearing
3. The retina is detaching.

A patch of lattice degeneration may atrophy slowly with insufficient disturbance of the surrounding retina to trigger spurious light impulses, and the resultant ring of spontaneous adhesion may have time to develop without the patient's being aware of anything untoward whatsoever. On the other hand, if the same patchy lattice is subject to traction, then points of light may wax and wane with each vitreal movement.

When the retina actually tears, the sudden loss of integrity is marked by a shocking and dramatic flash – rather like the beam of a lighthouse rotating to give acute intensity, then fading. The beam, however, only rotates once, because the mechanism causing the tear no longer exists once the retina has actually torn.

As the years pass, the quality of the vitreous (like that of any other body tissues) declines. It liquifies and collapses at random, with little lakes of fluid in its substance scattered like the holes in Emmenthaler cheese. As its inner structure weakens, the vitreous may detach from its normal position and separate from the retina, thereby disturbing it. The retina, true to its light-specificity, responds to this turmoil with shooting stars, each one replaced by another swooping into the darkness.

**Floaters**
When the neuroretina actually tears, the fragments of its substance (clumps of pigment or gushes of blood) spray into the vitreous as floaters, which then become the dominant symptom. Indeed, a haemorrhage can be so dominant that it obscures the vision totally, with a commensurate dulling of the red reflex.

Once the retina has begun to separate and the vitreous is clear enough to allow the patient to be aware of this separation, the curtain that veils the vision into blackness takes over from the floater. The very act of separation itself ruffles the photoreceptors into a glow like St. Elmo's fire, flickering constantly ahead of the advancing shadow.

Not all retinae detach so dramatically. A dialysis in the lower retina may take years to come to full flower. The retina detaches languidly, without any symptoms, until indolent field loss creeps close enough to the macula to be taken for a primary disturbance of central vision.


## EXAMINATION

Retinal examination begins like any other ophthalmic examination, with assessment of the central vision and the hand movement fields, followed by use of the slit lamp.

We can often be fooled by the patient's history, especially when a slow detachment in a phlegmatic individual is ignored or accepted as a lazy eye. Unexplained hypermetropic astigmatism should put us on the alert, and peripheral visual loss picked up by the hand movement field test can leave no doubt that the problem is retinal and not refractive.

The affected eye may give advance notice of detachment with a slight iritis and an intraocular pressure rather lower than that in the fellow eye and, significantly, blood or pigment debris in the anterior vitreous.

**Figure 4.2**
Uveitis, hypotony and an inverted umbrella detachment. A solemn warning not to offer surgery – first time or repeat.

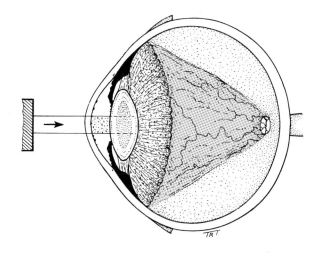

**Figure 4.3**
Retinal examination begins with the slit lamp. Vitreal detachment is not always as clear cut as this. A diagnosis of posterior vitreal detachment is made by the total absence of any signs that might explain the symptoms.

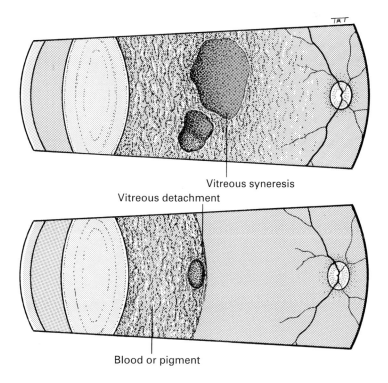

Vitreous syneresis

Vitreous detachment

Blood or pigment

Time, severity of detachment and unsuccessful surgery can all combine to damage the ciliary body. The uveitis may worsen and aqueous secretion decline – taking the eye to the point of collapse and shrinkage – if not immediately, then inevitably after further ill-advised interference in the name of treatment.

## State of the vitreous

A very degenerate (syneretic) vitreous betrays itself by large lakes of aqueous within its confines or by total collapse and detachment, when the posterior hyaloid with its ring of connection to the optic nerve may be detected parallel to the posterior surface of the lens.

Posterior vitreous detachment is a term that tends to be used casually to explain the existence of flashing lights and floaters when there is no detachment of the retina to account for them.

The normal vitreous with its languid undulating movements needs no description.

A rigid vitreous moves reluctantly with the eye, and returns quickly to its resting position. Such a vitreous is usually associated with evidence of traction on the surface of the retina, which does not augur well for the success of subsequent surgical intervention.

## Retinal examination

We all blithely talk of detachment as though the fundal appearance is never a source of doubt. The customary textbook clue of darkened blood vessels is a description of what is seen with difficulty with the direct ophthalmoscope when plus lenses are rotated into position. Using the indirect ophthalmoscope, such darkening is neither so apparent or so important.

The best sign of detachment is loss of the choroidal pattern behind a layer of subretinal fluid. This loss is best seen when moving from flat retina to detached retina, and the blurring of the pattern increases with increasing depth of subretinal fluid. It is important to remember, though, that when viewed through a thickened posterior capsule, all retinae have the spurious appearance of detachment.

It is pointless gazing at the retina in the hope that a break will eventually come out of hiding. The success of any fundal examination depends on knowing what we are going to find and where we are going to find it. After all, how many of us when assessing visual fields would find the blind spot if we did not already know where it was?

The form and distribution of a retinal separation in relation to the tear that gave rise to it are influenced by three naturally occurring factors:
1. Gravity
2. The anterior barrier of the ora serrata
3. The posterior attachment to the optic nerve head.

**Figure 4.4**
The critical sign of a detaching retina
is loss of the choroidal pattern.

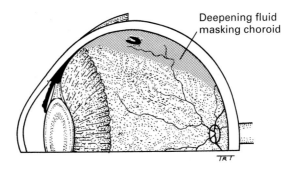

Deepening fluid
masking choroid

The progression, levels, contours and quadrants of the eye
favoured by the detachment depend on the position of the
primary retinal break, and *ipso facto* will lead an informed
observer to the correct location of the break.

There is a natural division of the upper retina into the
temporal and nasal halves by a vertical line rising from the
disc, which, although eccentric, is the 12 o'clock meridian. A
horizontal line divides the retina into the upper and lower
halves, cutting the disc along the meridians between 3 o'clock
and 9 o'clock, marked by the tramlines of the long posterior
ciliary vessels and nerves.

**Figure 4.5**
In the ocular clock face, the twelve
o'clock meridian lies directly above
the optic nerve head.

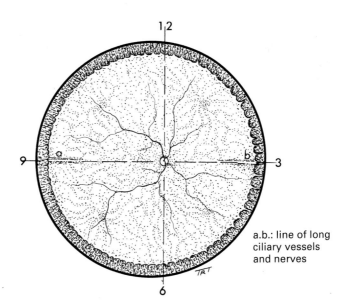

a.b.: line of long
ciliary vessels
and nerves

It is appropriate to consider the positions of retinal breaks
as map reference points, each break having two locating lines.
The first is the meridian conventionally described as hours of
the clock face, but each meridian also has another dimension
running backwards from the ora serrata to the optic nerve
head. Corresponding points on these meridians join up as

contour lines parallel to the ora serrata, giving every break
two points of reference:

1. A meridian
2. A contour line.

Subretinal fluid collects deep to the retina beside the major
break, and although a little fluid may creep upwards, by far
the greater portion tracks into the lower quadrants of the eye
under the influence of gravity. The higher the level of the
detachment, the higher the break must be.

**Figure 4.6**
Aphakic tears on different meridians
but on a common contour line behind
the vitreous base. This may be seen
after Yag capsulotomy and
extracapsular extraction with vitreal
loss.

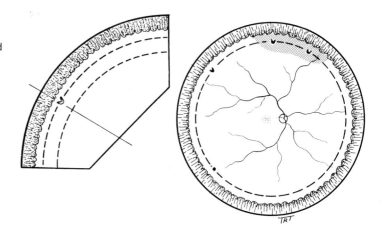

**Figure 4.7**
An upper temporal retinal
detachment. The first reference point
of the major break is the ten o'clock
meridian, the second is the contour
line corresponding to the equator.
Two further breaks on the same
contour line would remain
undetected unless looked for.

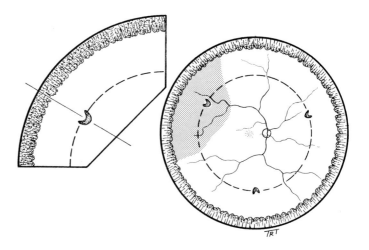

However, considering clock face meridians alone reduces
the ocular fundus to a flat surface, when quite clearly it curves
in three dimensions. The posterior segment is best imagined
as a brandy goblet lying on its side, with a curvature like the
side of an old wooden-walled battleship, making the diameter
of the ora rather less than the diameter of the equator. The
retina can then be imagined as kitchen clingfilm lining the
brandy glass, attached at the rim and at the stem.

**Figure 4.8**
The posterior cavity of the eye is like a brandy glass lying on its side, and the retina is like kitchen clingfilm attached at the rim and at the stem. In place of the brandy, there is a jelly attached at the rim and at the stem.

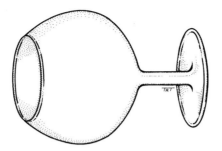

**Figure 4.9**
An inferior round hole; gravity and, possibly, a thick vitreous conspire to delay any awareness of this detachment until it catches the macula.

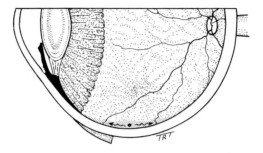

A break on a contour line running through the equator produces a detachment quite different from one that would follow a break beside the ora serrata. Subretinal fluid from an upper equatorial break quickly collects forwards towards the ora serrata, backwards towards the posterior pole and downwards on the contour line of the equator. Fluid from a lower equatorial break, on the other hand, rises slowly against gravity, forwards, backwards and to each side. With an upper oral break, subretinal fluid concentrates anteriorly to begin with, and tracks downwards along a line just behind the ora serrata before eventually spreading backwards. Subretinal fluid from a lower oral break (6 o'clock being the most extreme) spreads downwards and backwards to the equator before extending sideways. Knowing this behaviour, we can predict the position of retinal breaks before we find them.

**Figure 4.10**
An upper horseshoe break; gravity and the size of the break conspire to speed the development of this detachment. Symptoms of a field defect usually precede any macular involvement.

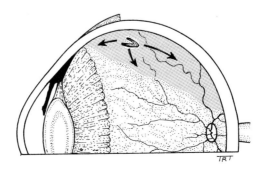

If a break is too small to allow free passage of formed vitreous, the separation of the neuroretina from the pigment retina will be slow enough to permit the creation of an inflammatory demarcation line. Such tide marks or high water marks occur in the shape of the advancing edge, but rarely manage to hold the detachment indefinitely. A series of these pigmented, retreating parallel defence lines – 'thin black lines' – form until the rising retina, catching the macula, can no longer be ignored. 'Tide rings', however, spontaneously encircling small round holes, tend not to need surgical assistance to keep the retina flat.

**Figure 4.11**
Gravity and the thick vitreous of youth allow the retina time to arrest its own detachment, in this case on three occasions, but on the fourth the detachment has burst sideways beneath the optic nerve head. The upper round hole could well have remained closed permanently. Large breaks always need surgery.

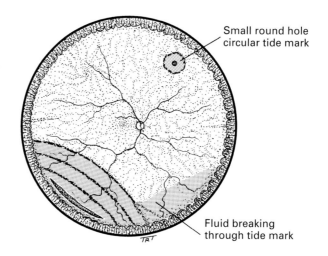

Small round hole circular tide mark

Fluid breaking through tide mark

It is part of retinal folklore that endless time spent in the darkroom before surgery will be rewarded with reduced time in the operating room. Such a belief, equating virtue with time invested, does not, alas, hold water. Indeed, it could well be that the length of the examination – in itself painful – could have been considerably reduced, had the surgeon known where to look for the retinal breaks in the first place. Undirected gazing into the eye will not discover salient features, but exposes the retina to needless light and raises fearful thoughts in the patient's mind about the surgical outcome, if the same struggle is to be duplicated in the operating room.

## UPPER BREAKS

The retina elevates around the break, and the elevation then spreads downwards on the side of origin. It continues around the lower edge of the disc and, if unchecked, rises up the other side. The higher level will always be found on the side with the retinal break and the higher the break, the higher will be the original level. Scleral depression, however, will always reveal a triangle of flat retina at 12 o'clock.

When the retinal break is near to the 12 o'clock meridian, this triangle disappears and the detachment spills over, descending on both sides of the optic nerve head until it finally becomes total. Rarely, sub-retinal fluid collecting from a hole at 12 o'clock may trickle down the ora serrata on both sides of the optic nerve head, filling out balloons in the lower quadrants of apparent equality, with neither side dominant.

**Figure 4.12**
The detachment is higher on the side with the break. A triangle of flat retina, straddling the twelve o'clock meridian, denies most detachments the description of 'total'. Subretinal fluid collection from a 12 o'clock break, however, will tumble down either side, favouring neither.

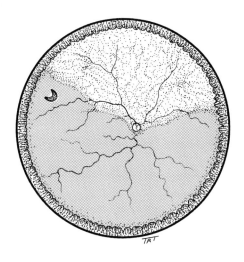

**Figure 4.13**
A multiple balloon detachment with a break at 12 o'clock. The retina at the posterior pole is relatively flat.

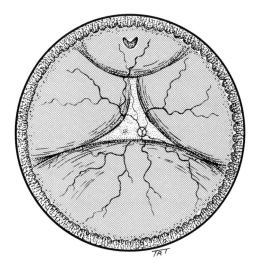

## LOWER BREAKS

When the retina is perforated below the horizontal meridian, the detachment behaves very much as one caused by an upper break except that all the signs occupy the lower quadrants, with the peccant break found on the side with the higher fluid level.

**Figure 4.14**
A lower temporal detachment with an equatorial horseshoe break. The fluid collection favours the side with the break.

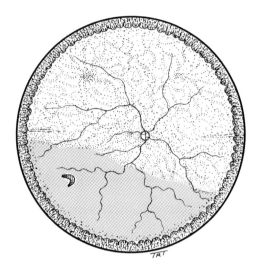

Should the opening in the retina centre on the 6 o'clock meridian, there will be no dominant level and the detachment bears a superficial resemblance to that caused by a tear on the 12 o'clock meridian.

The only factor that disturbs these simple principles is adhesion, produced either by trauma, spontaneous inflammation or previous surgery.

Lincoff and Gieser stated these principles definitively in 1971, but Gonin – the father of retinal surgery – published enough detail on the subject in 1934 to discredit the persisting belief that if the retina were gazed at for long enough, some essential sign would appear.

It should be remembered, however, that although the primary break may have its map reference point on a meridian and a contour line near the uppermost limit of a detachment, other breaks may lurk unsuspected in the detached – and often undetached – retina. A complete search must be made all the way round the contour line of the primary break (See Figure 4.7).

If the primary break has not revealed itself easily, it should also be remembered that the popular description of a retinal break as a red crack in a grey reflex has little basis in reality. The redness, when seen, depends entirely on how red the choroid is deep to the break, and if it can be viewed clearly. In breaks anterior to and beyond the equator, the choroid is more often stippled black and white, and more frequently still cannot be seen directly through a break. What can be seen, however, is a fragment (once part of an intact retina) wisping and floating from the retinal surface, rather like a goat's beard, and thrown into relief against the horizon by scleral depression.

As well as finding the break(s), the surgeon must also note the quality – whether the detachment quivers freely or lies immobile with rolled edges. A free, rippling detachment should flatten readily, whereas a motionless elevation with fixed star folds is already in the grip of preretinal retraction.

## BREAK NOT FOUND

Should skill and diligence still not discover the offending retinal defect, then a paracentesis, by allowing easier scleral depression in a softer eye, may uncover breaks that were formerly hidden in the shadows of one less easily indented.

**Figure 4.15**
A retinal break is red only if the underlying choroid is red. Peripheral tears are more commonly identified by the operculum, like a 'goat's beard', flung into profile by a scleral depressor.

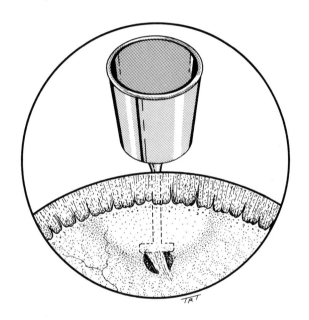

**Figure 4.16**
A rigid retina characterized by (1) continued traction on the operculum; (2) a break with rolled edges and (3) fixed star folds.

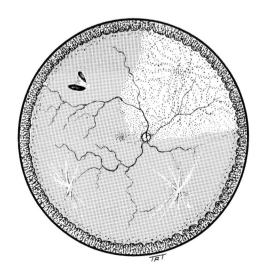

## VITREAL HAEMORRHAGE

Whilst most floaters appear as wisps or tendrils, a gush of blood into the vitreous (still theoretically described as floaters) will suddenly black out vision completely. If the patient cannot see out, the surgeon will have equal difficulty seeing in. Diabetes, hypertension, blood dyscrasias or trauma can all produce such a haemorrhage, but a hypertensive diabetic with a blood disorder or as a victim of trauma may still have a retinal detachment – a possibility rendered more likely by myopia, aphakia or a record of a detached retina in the past. Even the binocular indirect ophthalmoscope cannot pierce the mists of vitreal blood, but ultrasonic rays can, and are able to outline a fair imitation of what is happening deep in the cavity of the eye. B-scan ultrasound can trace the opacities, the thickness, the form and the behaviour of any membranes within the vitreal cavity. Any suggestion of a membrane fixed to the ora serrata and the optic nerve head must be taken to indicate the likelihood of a detached retina.

**Figure 4.17**
A funnel-shaped retinal detachment attached at the disc and at the ora serrata, and possibly obscured by haemorrhage. This would only be detectable by B-scan ultrasound examination.

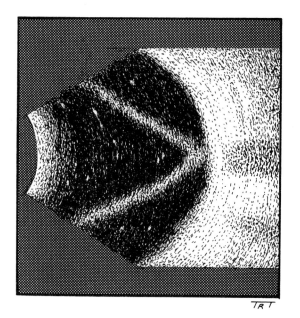

No examination is ever complete without close scrutiny of the fellow eye, in particular in the mirror image position, where similar disease might hide unsuspected pathology. In the case of trauma, there is no reason for the fellow eye to harbour mirror image change. Should it do so, the role of injury in the first eye might be less than was previously thought – a matter in which lawyers take great interest. A vulnerable retina detaching in response to minimal distur-

**Figure 4.18**
Eyes come in pairs. When one retina detaches, look at the mirror image position in the fellow eye.

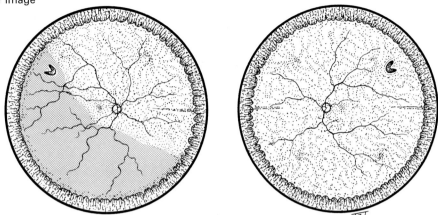

bance is legally very different from detachment of a normal retina after greater violence.

## REFERENCES AND FURTHER READING

Gonin, J. (1934). *Le Decollement de la Retine*. Payot Lausanne.
Lincoff, H. A. and Gieser, R. (1971). Finding the retinal break. *Arch. Ophthalmol.*, **85**, 565–569.

# 5

# Management of retinal detachment

Retinal detachment is only an emergency when the macula is intact or has just become detached within the previous 24–48 hours.

## SURGICAL MANAGEMENT

Although scientific support for it is weak, the preoperative application of topical antibiotics is a widespread practice – possibly doing as much good to the surgeon as to the patient.

The constant surgical aim is to reattach a functioning retina with a single procedure, and in such a way that a second procedure should prove unnecessary. In practice, this means making space within the eye to carry out the required manoeuvres without closing off the central retinal artery.

Operating on an eye with raised intraocular pressure not only further endangers the central retinal artery, but also threatens the catastrophe of an explosive incarceration of the retina during subretinal fluid release and raises the possibility of a clouding cornea when it is least wanted. It also goes without saying that any bleeding tendency, hypertension or diabetes should be noted and controlled to avoid increasing the risks to the patient and to the eye.

This surgery is best carried out under general anaesthetic, but retrobulbar anaesthesia (as for cataract surgery) will also serve the purpose. Preoperative sedation makes surgery easier for both patient and surgeon, and it should always be remembered that a gross manipulation apparently tolerated around the globe may fool us into thinking that the conjunctiva is equally insensitive when the time comes for closing up. The patient's distress on the operating table will very quickly remind us that it is not.

The pupil must of course be dilated with a combination of mydriatics, but if phenylephrine has to be used, application beyond the limbus will limit its damaging effects on the corneal epithelium. The epithelium can be further protected by forbearing to splash saline on the cornea from the beginning of the operation. This use of saline is another ritual lingering from the days of the direct ophthalmoscope, when the dominant fear was loss of a fundal view before surgery had properly commenced. Moistening the cornea too often and too soon will leach away the corneal lipids and bring about the very misting it seeks to avoid.

The cornea is most vulnerable to damage not only from instruments and from careless movement of the stay sutures, but also if the eyelids have remained open following the application of anaesthesia. Rather than struggle with an indifferent view, it is better to strip the epithelium completely and be aware that doing so will leave, at best, about 45 minutes in which to make out fundal detail essential for accurate surgery.

The conjunctiva should be opened at the limbus. Stay sutures are placed around the four rectus muscles, with particular care being taken not to catch the superior oblique along with the superior rectus muscle. Should the muscles prove elusive, it is helpful to catch each with one forceps before picking up the muscle edge with a second. It is important to remember that the sclera just deep to these muscles is relatively thin and vulnerable to perforation with the strabismus hook, and traction on the muscle should be relaxed just before the hook is inserted.

A suture of a different colour around the superior rectus will remind us to be constantly aware of how much torsion is being applied to the optic nerve. Torsion is not the only threat. If the passion to expose more sclera than strictly necessary makes us forget what connects the retina to the brain, we can proptose the eye outside the lids and add traction as well.

It is possible to bring a degree of swift elegance to all surgery by taking in further information whilst carrying out current procedures. For example, when the muscle sutures are being placed the sclera is visible, and examining it at this stage saves the need to check it later to determine the existence or extent of any dangerous areas of scleral thinning.

On commencing our search for the retinal break(s), a quick glance at the optic nerve head will tell us just how much pressure is required to make the central retinal artery pulsate. As we need to know this at some point, we might as well find out at the beginning. Indeed, knowing it may well stop us wasting time on one manoeuvre when the eye would clearly be happier with another.

In the search for the causal break(s) in the operating room, a round-tipped applicator is superior to the hammer head of the metal thimble depressor because it can be rolled around the eye with greater rapidity and accuracy. A moist cotton-tipped stick performs this role with ease, and has the added advantages of absorbing blood where it is not wanted and releasing any excess saline on the cornea before being

**Figure 5.1**
A plastic disposable glove, shapeless
but impermeable to bacteria, allows
the ophthalmoscope to be
manipulated during surgery. Use of
the glove on the right hand and the
covering paper in the left is a mild
gesture towards economy and a
significant one towards speed.

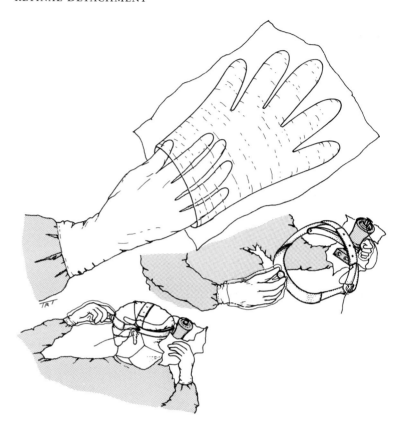

**Figure 5.1**
A plastic disposable glove, shapeless but impermeable to bacteria, allows the ophthalmoscope to be manipulated during surgery. Use of the glove on the right hand and the covering paper in the left is a mild gesture towards economy and a significant one towards speed.

deployed on the sclera. It is at this point that the value of good assistants becomes evident – either by their presence or by their absence. Quality support can do much to speed the operation along and increase the safety of its manoeuvres. It goes without saying that the sclera must be exposed and the blood mopped up, but more importantly still, the eye must be held firmly as the surgeon rolls a cotton-tipped applicator or applies a cryoprobe against the resistance of an immobile eye. The only person who can render the eye immobile is the assistant, and as with so many supportive actions, this excites maximal appreciation only when the help is not present. The assistant-induced immobility of the globe when activity on the sclera is being observed in the fundus cannot be emphasized enough, and it is one of the bedrocks of successful retinal surgery.

The essence of surgery can be summed up as follows:
1. Find all the breaks
2. Inflame the chorio/pigment retina where the breaks(s) will finally settle
3. Hold all the layers in contact until a watertight seal has formed
4. Prevent the break(s) from reopening.

**Figure 5.2**
The cotton-tipped applicator (1) absorbs blood; (2) rolls in any direction as a mobile scleral depressor; (3) maintains the intraocular pressure during hypotony, either expected or unexpected and (4) can moisten the cornea between examinations.

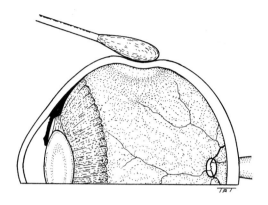

**Figure 5.3**
The rolling action of the scleral depressor. The retinal features are discovered only against resistance, and the assistant must hold the eye firmly, usually with the sutures around the twelve and six o'clock recti.

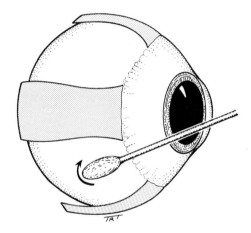

### How to find retinal breaks
The principles have been discussed in detail in the preceding chapter.

### The inflammatory insult
The technique currently in favour is a low temperature burn (cryopexy), applied through full-thickness sclera to that area of the choroid and pigment retina against which a break-bearing neuroretina is expected to form. If the neuroretina is already flat, then the freeze-burn whitens it as it spreads.

Laser photocoagulation is also popular but it can only be used when the retina is flat, except in certain circumstances where the beam can be delivered to the choroid and pigment retina deep to the break, usually during vitrectomy, with an endoprobe.

Breaks produced by trauma, particularly those with haemorrhage involving the choroid and pigment retina, already have a sufficient inflammatory insult to produce watertight scarring.

### Holding the layers together

Subretinal fluid release brings the layers together, but is not always necessary.

Internal tamponade with air or a mixture of air and gas seals the edges of the break(s) by surface tension, and floats the break(s) upwards against the inflammatory reaction.

Indentation of the ocular layers (scleral buckling) pushes the inflammatory reaction inwards towards the retinal break(s).

### Preventing the breaks from reopening

Scleral buckling may be sufficient as a permanent counter-traction. More persistent tractional bands can be removed with vitrectomy.

A common misconception fostered by examination questions is that there are discrete retinal operations, the use of one excluding the use of others. In fact, there is no such thing

**Figure 5.4**
Adhesion makes the tear watertight, and counter-traction keeps it so.

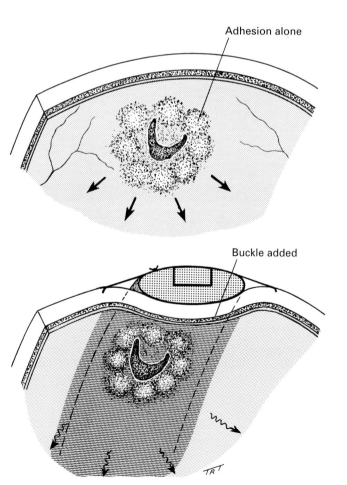

Adhesion alone

Buckle added

as any one single retinal operation, but rather a series of legitimate manoeuvres with which it is possible to carry out the aims of surgery. Many manoeuvres may achieve this end point. One or more might be necessary, but the final combination can only be guessed at before surgery. The final decision is best made by the eye itself, which will make it very clear during surgery which manoeuvres are favoured or will be tolerated. However, no one can argue with the notion that the best possible manoeuvre is the simplest that will achieve a permanent watertight seal without closing off the central retinal artery in the process, and without inflaming the eye so vigorously that a simple mobile detachment is turned into something rigid and untreatable instead.

A prerequisite for all retinal surgery is to warn the patient (in as comforting a manner as possible) that although nothing untoward is expected, a simple retinal detachment is one that is not yet complicated.

## LANDMARKS ON THE SCLERA

As details of the following techniques unfold, it will become apparent that callipers are one instrument with no place in the retinal tray. For too long, positions and movements about the sclera have been decreed by millimetre measurements based on a fictitious international standard eye. The location of the ora serrata and the equator vary like any other biological structure in their absolute position. Also, since the eye (like the world) is spherical, if millimetres are to be insisted upon, then they ought at least to be nautical millimetres. To state absolute measurements for the ora serrata and the equator and then to add or subtract a little makes a mockery of all millimetres, be they linear or nautical.

**Figure 5.5**
There is no international standard eye. The equator is always at the summit, but that summit is not the same distance from every limbus.

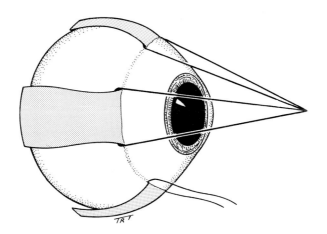

It is pointless to attempt to locate a deep structure by a measurement in surface millimetres, particularly when direct observation of this deep structure places it somewhere else. An obvious point that seems to be forgotten is that the deep structures, although varying in their absolute positions, have fixed and unvarying relationships to structures on the surface of the sclera. Since we can see these landmarks on the outside, we know the exact whereabouts of the related structures inside the eye that we cannot see.

### Ora serrata

The anterior limit of the retina – the ora serrata – lies deep to the rectus insertions and to the connecting furrow in the sclera produced by traction on the stay sutures. It is more anterior on the nasal than on the temporal side, and if any further surface indication is necessary, the sclera overlying the ciliary body differs markedly from that overlying the retina. First, its matted structure resists the easy passage of suturing needles, and secondly, the vascular network deepens as surgery progresses and ends abruptly at the line which connects the rectus insertions, marking very clearly where the retina ends and the ciliary body begins.

**Figure 5.6**
The ora serrata lies deep to the rectus insertions and to the small furrow produced between these insertions by traction on the stay sutures. Traction on these sutures may induce bradycardia.

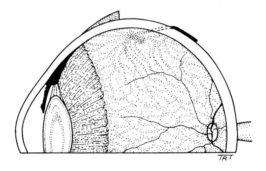

### Equator

The eye is a sphere. As the sclera continues backwards, it inclines to a summit and then begins to fall again into the depths of the orbit. This summit is the surface marking of the equator, and the vortex ampullae (as seen with the indirect ophthalmoscope) correspond to that contour line in the fundus.

The only possible contribution made by callipers is to increase the danger of perforating a thin sclera – a catastrophe doubly galling, since the manoeuvre that led to it was needless in the first place.

**Fig 5.7**
The sclera rises and then falls, and the summit – the point at which it does neither – marks the equator. This corresponds to the position of the vortex ampullae, and lies slightly anterior to the exit point of the actual vortex veins.

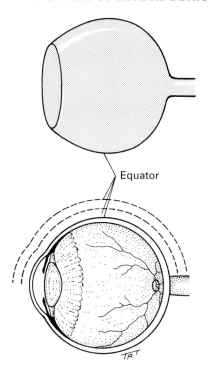

Equator

## Marking the sclera

If all features in the fundus were fixed in position, there would be no need to search for and mark their scleral equivalents. However, retinal breaks and fluid release sites by their very nature vary, and so we must be able to place marks over the surface relations that will last long enough to allow us to carry out any manoeuvres indicated with precision.

Many devices have been described, but the Gass locator must commend itself on the grounds of effectiveness, cost, and a total absence of moving parts that might go wrong. In essence, it is a scleral depressor with the crossbar removed

**Figure 5.8**
The Gass locator.

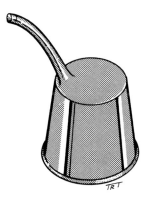

**Figure 5.9**
Gentle pressure with the locator at any selected point leaves a ring mark which is transient but useful. Marking this with a suture is certainly done, but marking it with a half-thickness sclerotomy designed for later use is both elegant and time saving.

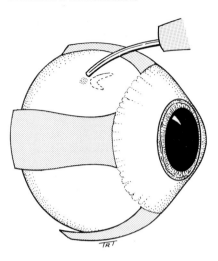

and the tip of the shaft fashioned into a blunt trephine. This tip is pointed enough to produce a precise and lingering mark on the sclera, but not so sharp that it might add a gratuitous wound of its own.

## CRYOPEXY

Cryopexy has replaced diathermy as the preferred method of the moment for applying an inflammatory insult to the chorioretina. The technique of manipulating the probe on the outside of the eye is merely an extension of scleral depression. The mound produced by such indentation can be seen easily with the indirect ophthalmoscope, and the probe positioned with great accuracy.

**Figure 5.10**
The freeze applications should be contiguous.

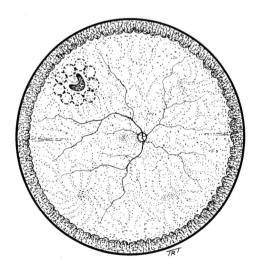

The applications must be contiguous. Each must be monitored, and the end point is the sudden appearance of an ice ball engulfing the retina. If the neuroretina is not in contact with the choroid the ice ball is not startlingly white, but rather a sudden spread of glazing in the choroid over the mound produced by the cryoprobe. Sometimes a glistening reflex is produced, and both these results are presumably the result of choroidal water turning into a convex ice mirror.

Just how long each application will take cannot be predicted in seconds. Each will vary with the strength of the cryo apparatus, the thickness of the sclera and the vascularity of the choroid, and the time may shorten even more as continued applications reduce the local temperature. It is for this reason, and not simply as a penitential exercise, that each application must be looked at.

**Figure 5.11**
The sudden appearance of an ice ball engulfing the retina is the sign to stop freezing at once. When the cryoprobe is not pressing directly over the retina, the sudden change of choroidal water into an ice mirror is not always obvious to the uninitiated. Timing a cryoapplication without observation is unacceptable.

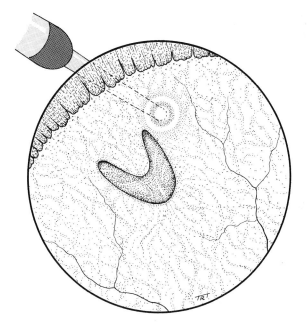

It is easy to forget that the act of pressing and freezing the eye raises the pressure of the eye beyond the pressure of the blood pumping through the central retinal artery. Patency of the artery can be preserved by the awareness that it is threatened. Certainly the probe has to be applied firmly to eliminate any fluid that might lie between its tip and the sclera and to produce effective freezing. However, once the freezing has begun, the pressure can be eased and the central retinal artery will begin to pulsate safely.

The practices of always turning the tip sideways to slide under the conjunctiva and of pressing away from the globe on entry reduce the risk of scleral damage and – in cases of extreme thinning – of scleral rupture.

If the area to be frozen lies in the extreme periphery, the adhesive qualities of the probe mean that it can be used as fixation forceps to turn the eye into a position that will allow its main use, as a freezing probe.

It is accepted as an axiom that cryopexy is rather like Robert Burns' 'snow fall on the river – a moment white and then gone forever'. This is not strictly true. Petechial haemorrhages on the sclera indicate exactly where cryopexy has been applied, and if the retina has been touched by the freezing, then cloudy patches of oedema can warn us where not to freeze again.

Although freezing has now supplanted diathermy as a method less likely to produce complications, particularly on the surface of the sclera, it does however carry certain risks within the eye. Cryopexy tends to dilate the blood vessels, weakening their walls and increasing the possibility of haemorrhage – a risk increased by excessive application, overly powerful cryo apparatus and, particularly, impatient removal of the cryoprobe before it has properly defrosted. In the more recent machines surgical impatience is not a problem because the probes defrost instantly, although sadly they do not always freeze as well as we would like.

It goes without saying that any bleeding tendency will be exaggerated by these low temperature activities.

Excessive freezing diminishes the very chorioretinal adhesion it seeks to bring about, and in its place brings atrophy of the ocular layers which in turn may lead to formation of further breaks in the retina.

A complication frequently linked with cryopexy, but happily less frequently seen, is disturbance of the pigment retina in a manner allowing scattered pigment to track downwards inevitably towards the macula.


## ENCIRCLEMENT


Despite popular belief, use of an encircling silicone band is not an operation in its own right. The translation of its name into French – *cerclage* – gives it an international flavour, and may well have obscured the fact that it is only part of a retinal operation. Memories of the old Arruga suture, which was strung around the eye as a new ora serrata and used as a substitute for finding retinal breaks (by giving the retina a new start whilst the old breaks remained untreated), together with anterior segment necrosis, have given the encircling band an unhappy and wholly undeserved reputation.

Reducing the diameter of the globe certainly slackens circumferential tractional forces, whilst displacing any formed vitreous backwards and forwards may well plug an open

**Figure 5.12**
The band is initially placed in contact with the globe just deep to the rectus insertions, and moving it from here to the equator creates the correct encircling tension. With the posterior limits of the suture in place, the thread is looped over and back under the band to allow placement of the anterior limb.

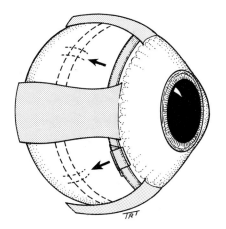

break. Silicone oil, if subject to the same anteroposterior displacement, may thus be effective with an encircling band. The uses of the band, however, go beyond these postulated advantages. It can keep guttered explants in position, readily becomes part of the sclera, and during surgery can be used to manipulate the position of explants without recourse to repeated scleral suturing.

To apply an encircling band, the 2 mm band (no. 40 in the MIRA catalogue) should be applied deep to the rectus insertions. Both ends should be tapered, but the tapering should be on one side of the band only; this subtlety allows us to observe whether the band has been twisted in its passage beneath the muscles. The ends are then joined by a Watzke sheath.

For some reason, this manoeuvre seems to cause endless problems, but need not. A 3 mm length of silicone sheath (inner diameter 0.76 mm, no. 270 in the MIRA catalogue) is slipped over the filed tips of a pair of mosquito forceps, the points of the forceps are then spread, and one end of the tapered band is fed through the sheath. The band is then slipped around the eye using the same mosquito forceps; starting at the lower nasal quadrant with one end, the other end will eventually make its way to the same quadrant. After pausing to make sure that the tapered edges taper on the same side, the modified mosquito forceps is insinuated between the sheath and the band, and the free end of the band is picked up with the tips of the forceps. This free end is then pulled through the sheath – an action facilitated if a thumbnail is used to hold the sheath back whilst the band is pulled through. The slack should then be taken up until the untwisted band just touches the globe deep to the rectus insertions. Casual pulling on the ends of the band increases the risk of twisting, and this can be avoided by holding the Watzke sheath with an untoothed forceps, much as a gun dog might hold game – firmly enough to secure, but not so tightly as to

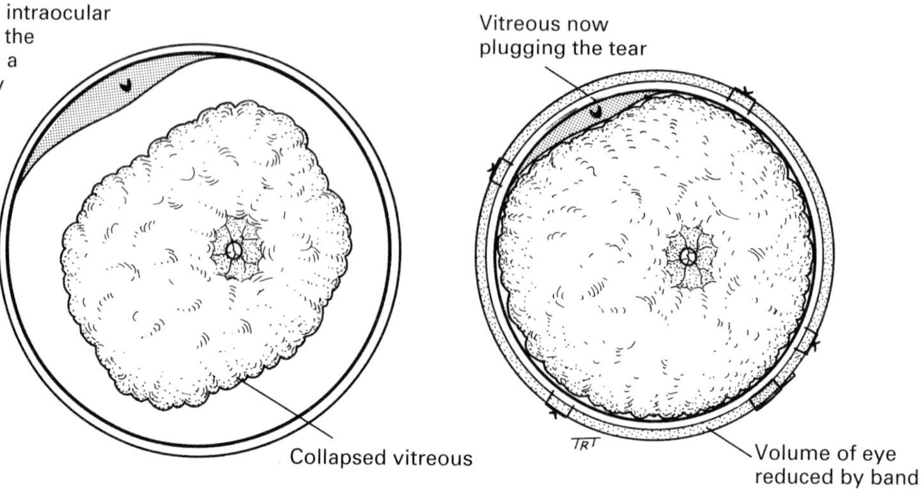

**Figure 5.13**
Encirclement is not an operation in its own right. It reduces intraocular volume, and may allow the formed vitreous to plug a break. It allows the easy manipulation of an encircling explant into place from the contour line and from meridian to meridian.

Vitreous now plugging the tear

Collapsed vitreous

Volume of eye reduced by band

damage. Care must be taken, because even if the bevels start correctly they do not always end correctly, and their positions should be observed after the band has been tightened. From this position, the band can be slipped back over the equator and sutured in place; here, its indenting force will be sufficient for all common detachments. Insertion of the first suture should be followed by its diagonal opposite (180° away) – this places the band in the final position and thus reduces doubts about the subsequent placement of scleral buckles.

**Figure 5.14**
A tapered mosquito forceps has many functions other than simple placement of the band.

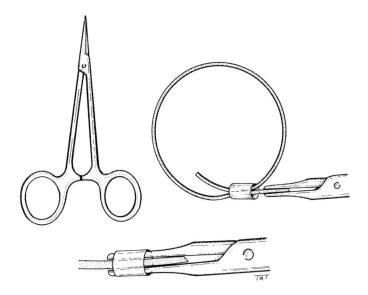

The silicone band has more tensile strength than can ever be used during a retinal operation, but it tears very easily when grasped with toothed forceps. These lacerations quietly deepen as the band is stretched, and if total rupture occurs, it tends to be when we are about to close up – an event trying for even the most phlegmatic of surgeons.

## SCLERAL EXPLANTS

The aim of the scleral buckle is to raise a mound in the ocular layers, thereby bringing the frozen area of chorioretina in particular into contact with the area of neuroretina bearing the break. The buckle should remain in position for at least long enough to allow the development of a watertight scar, and possibly indefinitely, to counter any tendency for the watertight scar to break open again (see Figure 5.4).

In the past, rival factions have debated the relative merits of radial and circumferential buckles. The argument against the radial buckle is that it causes asymmetric distortion of the globe, and that technically it is much harder to place a buckle on the correct meridian than it is to place one on the correct contour. The argument against the circumferential buckle is that by reducing the circumference of the equator, it throws the retina into redundant folds and one of these may run directly to the tear, producing the so-called 'fish mouth' phenomenon. The encircling band also produces a degree of myopia. As with all retinal manoeuvres, there is a place for each, depending on the eye.

### Radial sponge buckles

Silastic sponge comes in various shapes and sizes, with diameters ranging from 3–7 mm. Sponges tend to be bulky, and absorbed blood can provide a perfect culture medium for pathogenic micro-organisms; on the credit side, their pliant softness reduces the chance of scleral erosion.

To create a local buckle, the sutures must be tied under tension. They are, therefore, placed wide of the explant and

**Figure 5.15**
A bulky radial sponge beneath a rectus muscle may flatten the retina at the cost of double vision.

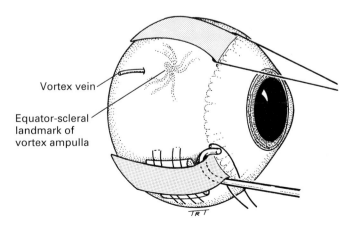

Vortex vein

Equator-scleral
landmark of
vortex ampulla

parallel to its long axis. Higher buckles and thicker explants demand wider suturing, and as a rough guide, the needle should enter the sclera at each side of the explant about half its width away.

A useful little buckle can be produced by tension-tying a 3 mm mattress suture without an explant. Combined with suitable photo- or cryocoagulation, this will often suffice for closing a small retinal tear – such as occurs when the scleral thickness has been misjudged and the retina pierced by a needle, or when the retina has been incarcerated during imperfect drainage of subretinal fluid.

**Figure 5.16**
Imbrication. A simple buckle without an explant. One throw followed by another in the same direction (using coated polyester) allows the knot to slide to the desired tension, and a throw in the reverse direction locks it permanently.

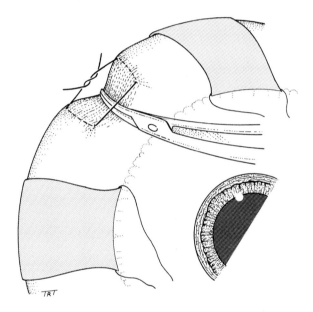

There is one further advantage to placing the suture tracks wide of the explant. If by chance the location of the tear has been less precise than it might have been, then it is useful to have some leeway on either side of the chosen meridian in order to seal the tear accurately.

### Circumferential explant

Although silastic sponge explants are made with gutters to accommodate the encircling band, the material favoured for this particular kind of explant is solid silicone rubber. These silicone explants come in a bewildering variety of shapes and sizes, and most of them derive their numbers from their original positions in the MIRA catalogue. They all offer qualities that might be preferable in differing circumstances, but two are sufficiently versatile to make the others unnecessary most of the time. These are the silicone strip (no. 20 in the MIRA catalogue), and the silicone tyre (no. 287 in the MIRA catalogue).

**Figure 5.17**
Equatorial horseshoe break treated with a radial explant, cryopexy and widely placed tension sutures. Meridians are harder to locate than contour lines, and a break missed in this way requires a completely new buckle.

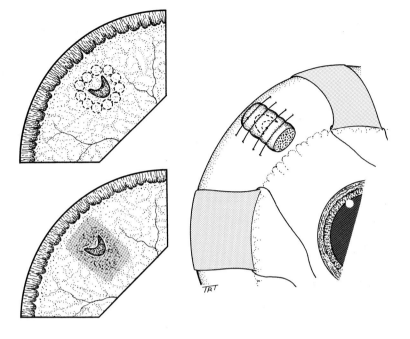

**Figure 5.18**
An equatorial horseshoe break. Treated using a circumferential explant band, widely placed tension sutures (for sutures, if tight is good, tighter is not necessarily better). There is more latitude for imprecision. The buckle may be moved sideways to a different meridian and the band may move the buckle to a new contour line; neither manoeuvre requires new tension sutures.

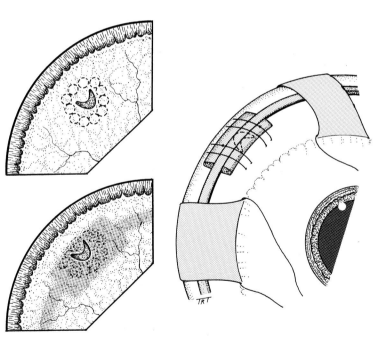

Any break must, of course, be located on the summit of the indentation rather nearer to its anterior edge. The same principles concerning suture placement apply, and rotating the knots to the posterior edge of the buckle reduces the amount of foreign material which may threaten to extrude through the conjunctiva later.

The great advantage of the circumferential explant is that there is far greater leeway for manoeuvre on a contour line than on a meridian, without the need for placing and replacing weightbearing sutures. These remain unchanged, and only the non-weightbearing holding sutures on the band need to be replaced. Holding sutures for the band do not require such security, and can be placed when the exact position is in mind.

**Figure 5.19**
Widely placed weightbearing sutures allow some leeway for manoeuvre, and sliding the explant along the band allows a correct meridian to be substituted for an incorrect one. Moving the band itself either towards or away from the ora serrata allows the already manoeuvrable explant to pick up the correct contour line.

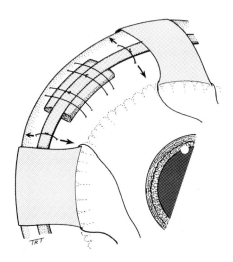

The disadvantage of redundant retinal folds and 'fish mouthing' need not be the problem suggested previously, and can generally be countered by injection of air into the vitreal cavity – a subject which will be explained later. However, the procedure should be extraocular if possible. An existing buckle can be augmented by placement of fragments of silastic sponge or of silicone rubber deep to it to fill any residual gaps between the retina and the indent. Should this fail, intravitreal air can be used without adding significantly to the length of the operation or to the manipulation of the eye.

### Subsequent exposure of scleral explants
The conjunctiva does not always share the desire that these buckles remain deep to itself, particularly when previous surgery has reduced its surface area. In such circumstances, conjunctival retraction exposes the explant, which in turn becomes a focus for recurrent discharge and infection.

Removal of the explant is one way to relax the conjunctival edges towards one another, but the explant was put there for a reason, which cannot simply be removed with it. An attempt can be made to suture the freshened edges of conjunctiva together, but unless traction is relieved by widespread dissection it will pull the edges apart again. In more extreme cases, a graft of buccal mucosa can fill the gap easily and is small enough to take its blood supply from adjacent freshened tissue. Donor mucosa can be taken from the inside of the lip adjacent to the lower teeth, and the defect closed with 7/0 polyglactin. Fat on the deep surface must be removed, and the graft (with the correct side outwards) is sutured to the freshened conjunctival edges with 8/0 poly- glactin on a spatulate needle. The graft should be twice the area of the gap being covered because it will shrink, and stretching a tiny fragment will merely duplicate the pathology that gave rise to the gap in the first place.

**Figure 5.20**
If the break remains open, a fragment of silastic sponge deep to the buckle may seal it without recourse to further scleral sutures.

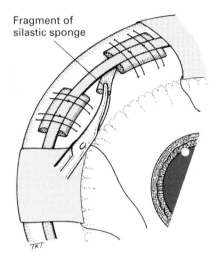

Fragment of silastic sponge

## TECHNIQUE OF SUTURING

These buckles would all be pointless unless stitched on in such a way that they do not slacken easily, and without per- forating the retina with the suture needle.

Various materials can be used for suturing, but certain qualities raise polybutylate-coated polyester above its rivals. The 5/0 gauge is strong enough for any level of tension sutur- ing, the material slides easily through the sclera, and whilst two throws in the same direction allow the knot to slide to the desired tension, one throw in the reverse direction locks the knot permanently. None of these qualities is of any use, how- ever, if the needle does not allow the suture to be placed in the sclera alone, without damaging the retina. A half-circle (5/8) spatulate needle permits manipulation behind the equator, and moderate sharpness remaining uniform throughout the operation is infinitely preferable to razor sharpness, which may create problems initially, and again later when bluntness increases the pressure required to make any impact at all on the sclera.

It is assumed for some reason that every surgeon knows instinctively how to insert these needles. This may be because most young ophthalmic surgeons are blooded on strabismus surgery, on the assumption that it is somehow safe. However, the danger of retinal perforation then is as great as during retinal surgery, and only the thickness of the young vitreous prevents embarrassment later.

The steps to correct suturing are as follows:

1. Hold an adjacent rectus insertion with fixation forceps to tether the eye
2. Dimple the sclera with the needle tip to the desired depth
3. Advance the needle through the scleral lamellae with the back surface of the needle leading and the tip pointing away from the retina.

There are two concurrent motions; the needle rotates on its axis like a wheel, and the whole complex moves gently forwards at the same time. The motion is not unlike that of the prow of a boat rising and dipping in the water.

Although the aim is to place a stitch that will not cut out of the sclera, it is equally important that it should not cut into the retina. In trying to avoid retinal perforation, there is a strong temptation to drag the needle away from the sclera rather than using the correct technique, which is to control the needle's passage along the sclera. All surgeons go too deep from time to time and the sensation is unmistakable, with the needle moving into an empty void and nothing to steady its tip – or the nerves of the surgeon – at the other end. Any such perforation has the matchless advantage that we know exactly where it is, and treatment is usually achieved by cryopexy and either by altering the position of the buckle slightly or by internal sealing with an air bubble.

**Figure 5.21**
The essential technique of scleral suturing. The sclera is dimpled to the correct depth with the back and the tip of the needle, and the needle (now parallel to the scleral lamellae) is driven to the selected depth, always presenting its safe surface to the retina. The needle is rotated on its own axis like a wheel whilst moving gently forwards at the same time. The temptation to drag the needle away from the sclera and retina must be resisted.

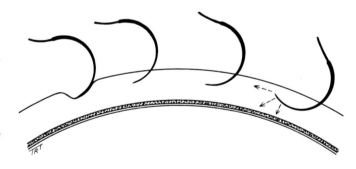

## INTRAVITREAL AIR

A bubble of air injected into the vitreous will seal the edges of a break floated on its summit by surface tension, and this is an easy and effective way to place the edges of large, irregular, ragged tears against the frozen chorioretina. These edges tend to follow the contours of the globe, and because of this they are much more likely to adhere in this position than when draped over the unnatural hump of a large buckle.

At repeat operations, intravitreal air vastly reduces the complexity of buckling sclera that may well have been so manipulated in the past as to make further buckling impossible. Predictably, for many years there were several popular misconceptions about the use of air, but happily these are no longer believed. It does no harm to mention them, however.

There is a general belief that air obscures the retinal view. This is not true, except when multiple bubbles are scattered like frogspawn through the anterior chamber of an aphakic eye, and not always then. Tapping the eye with a finger or a cotton bud encourages multiple bubbles to coalesce into a single larger one, and indeed they may do so spontaneously in time. The view through the bubble is improved further by indentation of the retina under scrutiny. It also used to be widely stated that air did not last long enough to seal a retinal break. This is just not true; twelve hours may be long enough.

A single bubble can always be produced with one movement of the plunger of a dry syringe and a dry needle passed through the pars plana anterior to the rectus insertion. It is sometimes easier to see through this bubble than through the natural vitreous, which may well be obscured by blood and other debris.

If the major surgical manipulation is over, then the intraocular pressure can be normalized. If however further buckling or other action is required, then leaving the eye slightly softer than normal will create enough space for the procedure.

If the subretinal fluid has been released in the vicinity of a retinal break, then the air will bubble out freely unless the sclerotomy is tightly closed.

**Figure 5.22**
The injecting needle is passed through the sclera and the pars plana anterior to the rectus insertions, and therefore anterior to the ora serrata. A single movement of a dry plunger with a dry syringe and dry needle will produce a single bubble.

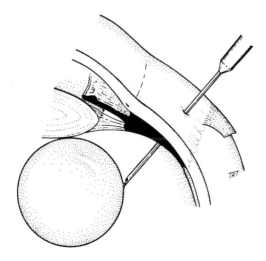

**Figure 5.23**
An air bubble seals by surface tension
and not by pressure.

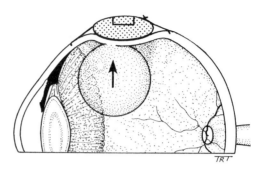

The major disadvantage of air is that it converts what might be an extraocular procedure into an intraocular one, with the potential danger of intraocular infection. This danger must be balanced against the possibly greater danger of leaving the retina sterile, but still detached. A second disadvantage is the technical difficulty of injecting air into a soft eye. The air may be needed in a hurry to make up the ocular volume, but the eye may be too soft to allow the needle through the pars plana. Forcing the needle against resistance may strip the pars plana and hit the lens. This problem can sometimes be circumvented by holding a rectus muscle firmly in the fixation forceps, and introducing the needle just anterior to the insertion. Third, the needle (if not clearly into the vitreal cavity) will liberate the air deep to the neuroretina, or into the suprachoroidal space. If necessary, this ectopic air can be released in the same way as the subretinal fluid. A fourth disadvantage, although essentially a careless disaster, is closure of the central retinal artery.

The subtlety in refined surgery is to make observations that do not appear initially to have any apparent relevance. The speed of postoperative disappearance of an air bubble can tell us a lot about the intraocular pressure. Rapid absorption of a large bubble means that the pressure is high, and conversely, languid absorption indicates that it is low.

### Anaesthetics and bubbles

If nitrous oxide ($N_2O$) is favoured by the anaesthetist this must be turned off 30 minutes before the intravitreal air is injected, for two very significant reasons:

1. During general anaesthesia, the high concentration of nitrous oxide ($N_2O$) displaces nitrogen ($N_2$) in the air bubble. This causes a potential dangerous expansion of the bubble, threatening the central retinal artery
2. Conversely, when $N_2O$ disappears from the blood later on it also disappears from the eye, converting the danger of a large bubble into that of a small bubble.

### Other gases

The numerous advantages of air led naturally to the desire for something even better, which would remain longer within the vitreal cavity. Sulphorhexafluoride (SF$_6$) was the first gas (popularized by Norton) to offer this quality, but there are others, each with a special claim, such as Perfluoropropane (C$_3$F$_8$). Such an additional quality comes at a price. These gases attain their long presence in the eye by expanding, and expansion threatens to close the central retinal artery. SF$_6$ expands to twice its volume over 12–18 hours, whilst C$_3$F$_8$ expands more slowly (over 24 hours) to three times its original volume. Apart from the perils of expansion, the mere presence of these gases in prolonged contact with the crystalline lens will produce a cataract – transient, but usually still present when the surgeon is trying monitor the effect of the previous day's operation.

In routine surgery involving intravitreal air, mixtures with 20% SF$_6$ and 12% C$_3$F$_8$ prolong the effect of the bubble without any attendant danger to the central retinal artery. The mixture can be made up in a syringe in advance and, needless to say, there are instruments which will deliver the appropriate concentration automatically.

These gases have other dangers which will be discussed under pneumatic retinopexy.

## SUBRETINAL FLUID RELEASE

Another reflex is the division of retinal surgeons into those who release fluid and those who do not. Here we find yet another example of a controversy that should now belong in the pages of a closed book, but which has persisted as a surgical divide. To release or not to release is not a question of incompatible beliefs. If fluid needs to be released then it should be released, and if release can be avoided then it should be, but not if avoidance exposes the eye to greater danger.

We should recognize that a detachment is only as deep as that area bearing the retinal break. This area can often be remarkably shallow despite the presence of great balloons of detachment that almost touch in the mid cavity of the eye. Such knowledge is critical, because it is the break we treat and not the rest of the retina.

The criteria for releasing subretinal fluid are met in four definite circumstances:
1. When the manoeuvre selected requires more space than is available.
2. When the retinal break is too widely detached from its chorioretinal bed to allow accurate application of the cryoprobe, or if with a local buckle it is impossible to know precisely where the tear is going to settle. By persisting with cryopexy when neither the tip of the probe nor

**Figure 5.24**
A detachment is only as deep as that part of the retina bearing the retinal break. Subretinal fluid does not require to be removed just because it is there – treatment must be directed at the break. Watching the fluid disappear is more comforting than waiting for it to come back.

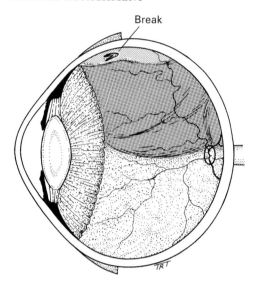

the end point can be identified, the surgeon may be tempted to try excessive freezing as a substitute for accurate freezing. Occasionally, the act of applying the cryoprobe may induce the subretinal fluid to become more shallow but this should not be counted upon.

3. When in any longstanding detachment (particularly those associated with dialysis or disinsertion) the neuroretina is invariably separated from the underlying pigment retina and choroid by extremely thick subretinal fluid. Any attempt to buckle such a break without prior fluid release will simply result in a procession of all the ocular layers, still defiantly separated, towards the centre of the eye.

4. When a rigid deep detachment demands a high buckle that on its own would close the central retinal artery. Such an

**Figure 5.25**
Subretinal fluid release is obligatory when (1) the detachment is too deep for accurate cryopexy; (2) thick subretinal fluid lies deep to dialysis of disinsertion; (3) we need to make space or (4) a rigid retina requires extra buckling.

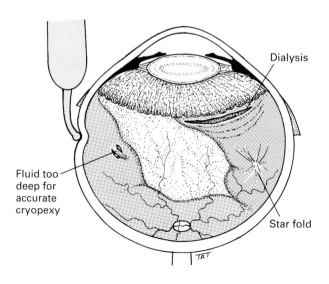

eye can sometimes be softened adequately with prior release of subretinal fluid, but if adequate space cannot be created from beneath the retina then of course vitrectomy is required to make space in the vitreal cavity.

Rules about release of subretinal fluid can be traced back (like so much else in retinal surgery) to the days of the direct ophthalmoscope. These former rules recommended that the drainage site should never be cut midway between the rectus muscles for fear of rupturing the vortex veins. The vortex veins do tend to leave the sclera midway between the muscles, but the vortex ampullae (the parts we are trying to avoid) remain within the eye, and possibly on a meridian which the old rules considered to be safe. However, their contour line can invariably be taken as a landmark for the equator.

### Where to release subretinal fluid

In the past, there was as much disagreement about where fluid should be released as about when and if it should be released. Some surgeons preferred release anterior to the buckle and some posterior, although all agreed that a point directly over a retinal break should be avoided.

Fluid release directly over a break does, however, bring with it certain advantages:
1. The retina is already torn and therefore cannot suffer further damage at this point
2. A precise scleral surface landmark for the retinal break is provided
3. Subretinal fluid flows selectively from the subretinal space, whilst formed vitreous (if any should be present) remains within the vitreal cavity. If 'fluid' vitreous is escaping, then we can allow this to continue until enough space is made for the manoeuvre selected. The intraocular pressure should be maintained by injection of air into the vitreous before extreme softening of the eye makes injection impossible.

It would appear then that the obvious place to release fluid is where there is fluid already, and that, not unusually, is where the retina is torn. However, the presence of large choroidal vessels in the area must lead us to a site where the choroid is less vascular.

### Technique

The first step is to locate the exact point on the sclera considered safest for the release of the subretinal fluid. Then, with the eye firmly tethered, an incision is made in the sclera at right angles to the ora serrata. The incision is then deepened until a knuckle of black choroid gleams in the depth of the sclerotomy. Cautery to this knuckle dulls its gleam, indicating that the choroidal blood flow is sufficiently diminished to allow us to perforate it with a fine-tipped needle (outside the eye) without causing haemorrhage inside the eye.

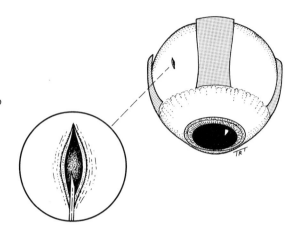

**Figure 5.26**
Subretinal fluid release. (1) This should be carried out where there is subretinal fluid. (2) The choroid must be relatively avascular. (3) The choroid is cauterized. (4) The perforating needle does not dip through the choroidal knuckle deep to the scleral surface.

Although tradition always recommends suturing of the sclerotomy site, this is necessary only in two circumstances: first, to prevent intravitreal air bubbling out through a scleral incision directly over a retinal break; or secondly, when it is anticipated that a scleral buckle is going to raise pressure in the eye at the risk of expelling the retina through the fluid release site.

It is anticipation as much as care that prevents needless disasters. Sudden collapse of the intraocular pressure may lead to suprachoroidal bleeding, but it is more likely to lead to cataract. Such dangers can be obviated by having ready some method of restoring the intraocular pressure to an acceptable level. This may be injection of air into the vitreal cavity, or by having any tension sutures associated with a buckle already placed and ready to tie. Prior to either solution, constant pressure with a cotton-tipped applicator guards against hypotony.

### Incarceration

The retina can be trapped in the sclerotomy if the fluid is not deep and the intraocular pressure is high. Occasionally during surgery the pressure may be raised by external manipulation. Bulging of the choroid warns us to be on our guard, and a paracentesis at this point will reduce the intraocular pressure sufficiently to allow us to carry out our intended course of action safely.

Should disaster strike in the form of an incarceration (as it must at some time to every one of us) then at least we know the whereabouts of the potential perforation. This must be treated as any other perforation, with cryopexy and a local buckle, on the assumption that some local traction elements may develop later.

### An old technique resurrected

It was common practice for many years to make multiple punctures of the sclera, using a guarded catholysis needle, into what was hoped to be a reservoir of subretinal fluid. Although the electrically-based system was reasonably expected to limit choroidal bleeding, the manoeuvre acquired an unfortunate reputation for puncturing the retina instead – mainly because of poor site selection. Provided we can see where the deepest well of fluid exists, it is perfectly acceptable to perforate into this with the same needle used for buckle suturing. 2 mm of needle protruding from a needle holder guarantees the same depth of penetration into the subretinal space each time. This may need to be reduced for a very thin sclera. The resultant flow is languid and therefore demands a degree of patience, but it also gives the surgeon time to respond to untoward events.

### To release or not to release

Not all the subretinal fluid has to be released. The aim is to make space so that certain manipulations are possible. It is not necessary to make the retina look attractive on the operating table, and indeed it is more comforting and informative afterwards to watch the fluid disappear than to wait for it to come back.

The controversy surrounding the release of subretinal fluid would not have arisen were the manoeuvre totally without complications, which of course it is not. Most of the dangers that threaten can be avoided with a little foresight.

A raised intraocular pressure – unusual in the presence of a retinal detachment – can sweep the retina into the release site sclerotomy. Even if pressure is normal, a similar disaster can follow attempted release where the fluid is too shallow.

It is unreasonable to expect cautery or diathermy to check the flow of blood through the large choroidal vessels, and careless site selection will result in haemorrhage in all directions.

The knuckle of choroid should be perforated with a needle as its convexity presents in the depth of the sclerotomy. Should the expected subretinal fluid fail to materialize, digging into the cavity of the eye will not make it do so. It may however perforate the retina, producing vitreous in place of subretinal fluid and haemorrhage, adding to our anguish.

Tapping a deep balloon of subretinal fluid may sometimes cause something like an oil well that will not stop gushing. Unless precautions are taken, the inevitable result is a soft eye. Such precautions might include pre-placement of tension sutures to be tied over the relevant buckle, or an air syringe held in readiness to restore the intraocular pressure to soft normal. Failure to protect the eye against collapse of intraocular pressure may (particularly in the elderly) result in intraocular haemorrhage, damage to the lens and suprachoroidal effusion.

Trying to place tension sutures in an eye where the normal scleral convexity is softened out of shape will result either in shallow placement that will only cut out under tension, or in too deep a placement that will almost certainly perforate the retina, rendering the chosen buckle useless.

Another danger with the soft eye is the temptation to make up the volume by excessive buckling, and it is wiser to resist the temptation at the operating table than to regret it the following day. The disruption of the barrier of the internal limiting membrane and of the walls of the retinal vessels can lead to proliferative vitreoretinopathy, and if the vitreous itself presents in the wound, transglobal traction bands contracting with time will increase the tendency to detach. However, a slightly softened eye and a temporary suture to prevent continued flow from the fluid release sclerotomy does make scleral depression easier, which in turn makes for easier discovery of as yet unfound retinal breaks.

## PARACENTESIS

Maintaining the patency of the central retinal artery must always take precedence over any of the surgical manoeuvres which threaten it. If space cannot be made for the necessary surgical replacement of the retina by subretinal fluid release, then another way must be found to reduce the pressure of the eye sufficiently to allow the manoeuvres to be carried out in safety. If the anterior chamber is reasonably deep – and in most cases it is – then recurrent tapping for aqueous is a very useful way of bringing the intraocular pressure down sufficiently to allow a buckle to be tied under tension or air to be injected into the vitreous cavity whilst maintaining the patency of the central retinal artery. The constant production

**Figure 5.27**
Patency of the central retinal artery must take precedence over all other factors. If subretinal fluid has not been released, it may be threatened by cryopexy, air injection or excessive buckling. The 'feel' for its collapsing pressure should be noted at the beginning of the operation, and its patency must be demonstrated by direct observation at the end of surgery.

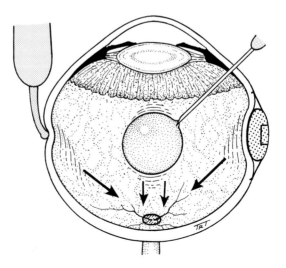

of aqueous refills the anterior chamber, and the new level of intraocular pressure must be maintained. Repeated release of the aqueous through the same opening is as simple as it is effective. The technique is to introduce an angled blade – the sharper the better – at the limbus, whilst holding an adjacent rectus insertion firmly. If however the eye is already soft, any attempt to make it softer still by paracentesis will fail, because aqueous will only flow from the anterior chamber if the intraocular pressure is normal or raised.

It is unhappily at such times, when we need a particularly good view of the fundus, that the pupil will decide to respond to hypotony with constriction.

**Figure 5.28**
Paracentesis – a vital manoeuvre in making space. The knife must be sharp, the entry wound must be free of limbal vessels and the blade must be parallel to the iris surface. Fluid will not flow from the anterior chamber unless the intraocular pressure has been slightly raised by, for example, air injection. The opening may be tapped at regular intervals.

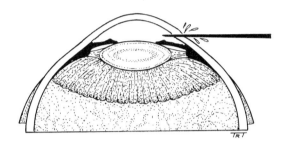

To avoid pitfalls:
1. The blade must be razor sharp to allow unhindered passage into the anterior chamber
2. Tethering an adjacent rectus muscle permits the blade to be introduced with controlled pressure
3. The handle should move freely without lodging against any possible impediment that could suddenly give way as pressure is increased, thereby causing the blade to make high-speed contact with the lens.

### Making space following vitrectomy
In the unhappy event of a redetachment following vitrectomy, space can be made by removal of the now liquid vitreal contents through the pars plana. The technique is simple. A 25 gauge needle attached to a 2 ml syringe is passed into the vitreal cavity, monitored with the indirect ophthalmoscope if required. The fluid volume appropriate to the space desired is withdrawn. Should intravitreal air be indicated, then an air syringe can be attached to the same needle, left *in situ*, after the first syringe is detached.

### Aphakic eyes
Occasionally, a shallow anterior chamber makes paracentesis impossible. Particular care should be taken in eyes that have undergone intracapsular extraction. Vitreous may not start in the anterior chamber, but the passage of aqueous may drag it

forwards and indeed into the limbal opening. Vitreous lost in this way will often increase the depth of the retinal detachment, but this is the price we must pay for not being able to release subretinal fluid. Provided the tears have been sealed and prevented from reopening by sufficient counter-traction, the slight delay in absorption of subretinal fluid will turn out to be very little cost at all.

Vitreal strands stretching into the corneal puncture wound are best removed with a vitreous suction cutter. If this had been used to make space to begin with, it may well not be needed now. The ocular volume can be preserved during this exercise with the anterior chamber maintainer.

## SUMMARY

Such then are the techniques available to treat most retinal detachments. It is worth repeating that there is no such thing as a single retinal operation. We should approach the eye with some idea of what we would like to do, but must always be prepared to abandon it if the eye clearly demands an alternative.

In the approach described in this book, cryopexy is the only obligatory manoeuvre, although the encircling band is also favoured. Thereafter, any operation becomes a selection of the simplest manoeuvres that will flatten the retina without closing the central retinal artery. We must make space in the eye to do what has to be done and no more.

If the retinal tear is shallow, then it might be possible to catch this tear with a circumferential buckle alone. If the central retinal artery is threatened, then a paracentesis might restore its patency. It should be remembered that an encircling band is already a threat to the central artery; if it becomes clear that this simple manoeuvre alone is inadequate, then it is pointless rediscovering the obvious during time that could have been better spent on a more radical procedure. It may well be that fluid must be released, and if this is the case, the first step is to reduce the intraocular pressure by cutting the tension sutures on the buckle. Fluid can then be released as described. It is critical to anticipate a copious flow with a ready air syringe or a preplaced tension suture. If the buckle is still not catching the tear as we would like and we are satisfied that it is in the correct position, then the buckle may be augmented with an injection of air into the vitreous.

By approaching each detachment flexibly in this way, it is possible to tailor-make the operation to meet the demands of every eye.

## CLOSURE

It is at this point that we find again how difficult it is to anaesthetize the conjunctiva with local anaesthetic. A single stitch on the temporal side of the globe is enough to bring its edges together, deliberately leaving a 2 mm gap around the limbus. Although it might appear tempting to fill this gap with conjunctiva at the end of the operation, doing so will cover the cornea with conjunctiva the day after.

In many centres it is customary to inject solutions of antibiotic and corticosteroid into the conjuctiva. The swelling so caused is but a small price to pay for the increased speed with which all swelling settles later, and it does not obscure the cornea during postoperative examination.

It should not be necessary during any of the foregoing techniques ever to detach an extraocular muscle. Exposure is not improved and a vital landmark is lost, whilst in its place comes the threat of anterior segment ischaemia followed by the ultimate mortification when the patient's gratitude over a flat retina is tempered by persistent double vision.

Approaching an eye in this way allows great flexibility and relieves worry over the correctness of a procedure. All procedures are potentially correct, and if we offer one that the eye seems to accept, then it is highly likely that we will have chosen the right one.

## POSTOPERATIVE CARE

Postoperative care is simple. The eye's response to interference is a generalized inflammation and possibly iritis, and topical corticosteroids over the first two or three weeks will reduce this inevitable inflammation. Mydriatics such as cyclopentolate keep the iris mobile and allow postoperative examination. A single pad will protect the eye until it stops watering; bilateral pads only depress the patient. They doing nothing to reduce the mobility of the eye, a former aim which is of questionable value anyway, and more to the point, they give the patient the foretaste of what may lie in store for them should both retinae detach and all operations fail.

If subretinal fluid has been released, we must look to see if it is returning. If it has not been released, we gain even greater pleasure in observing its departure. Fluid absorption may be slow in long-standing detachments, and this in itself is not an indication to reoperate immediately. Provided the retinal break is flat and 'dry' on the buckle and on the encircling band, we should be prepared to wait and observe the patch of fluid that is being slowly absorbed. If on the other hand the collection deepens, then we have to look for a source.

Follow-up will depend on many factors both social and economic. In the short term, we are concerned about intra-ocular infection and the successful outcome for our surgical aims. In the long term, we are more concerned with any possible ill effects of our manoeuvres – whether a tight band is eroding the sclera or an explant being extruded. Any hint that the choroidal pattern is disappearing again is a signal to begin the search for another retinal break at the upper border between normal and flat retina.

It is often quietly forgotten that attached to a successfully treated detachment is a patient who will meekly await instructions to return to work. The wait may be unnecessarily long if the surgeon thinks only of the retina and the patient hesitates to ask for fear that normal daily activity will be permanently banned. The resumption of normal life should be complete after a maximum of four weeks. Clearly, this does not mean total inertia followed by total mobility, but rather a gradual increase to peak performance, as happens when a car is being run in. The only embargo might be on violent contact sports, particularly those involving impacts to the head, but if the patient happens to be a footballer or a boxer such recommendations might not carry the weight that they would to others.

Once the eye has recovered from the physical assault of surgery, there is nothing to gain from a six- or twelve-monthly follow-up examination. If the retina is going to detach again, then it will do so regardless, and if so it is often from a lesion that could never have been predicted. It also usually seems to occur just after the most recent visit!

## REFERENCES AND FURTHER READING

Custodis, E. (1960). Scleral buckling without excision and with polyviol implant. In *Importance of the Vitreous Body with Special Emphasis on Reoperations* (C. L. Schepens, ed.) pp. 175–182. Mosby.

Charles, S. T. (1985). Controlled drainage of subretinal and choroidal fluid. *Retina*, 5, 233–234.

Chawla, H. B. (1970). A new instrument for use in retinal detachment surgery. *Br. J. Ophthalmol.*, 54, 494.

Chawla, H. B. and Birchall, C. H. (1973). Intravitreal air in retinal detachment surgery. *Br. J. Ophthalmol.*, 57, 60–70.

Chignell, A. H. and Talbot, J. (1978). Absorption of subretinal fluid after non-drainage retinal detachment surgery. *Arch. Ophthalmol.*, 96, 635–637.

Chignell, A. H. and Wong, D. (1986) The role of induced choroidal retinal adhesion in retinal detachment surgery. *Trans. Ophthalmol. Soc. UK*, **105**, 580–582.

Gass, J. D. M. (1966). A scleral marker for retinal detachment surgery. *Arch. Ophthalmol.*, **76**, 160.

Gonin, J. (1930). The treatment of detached retina by searing the retinal tears. *Arch. Ophthalmol.*, **4**, 621–625.

Lincoff, H. A., Baras, I. and McLean, J. M. (1965). Modifications to the Custodis procedure for retinal detachment. *Arch. Ophthalmol.*, **73**, 160–163.

McLeod, D. (1986). Fresh retinal detachments – the role of scleral buckling. *Trans. Ophthalmol. Soc. UK*, **105**, 480–488.

Michels, R. G. (1986). Scleral buckling methods for rhegmatogenous retinal detachment. *Retina*, **6**, 1–49.

Schepens, C. L., Okamura, I. D. and Brockhurst, B. J. (1957). The scleral buckling procedures. 1. Surgical technique and management. *Arch. Ophthalmol.*, **58**, 797–811.

# 6

## Putting the manoeuvres into practice

*Best is the enemy of good* – Voltaire

Do not deliberate over decisions already made; good is the enemy of perfect. However we phrase it, the message is clear; if the retinal position at the end of an operation is acceptable, we must not spoil it by trying for absolute perfection.

Surgery and golf have many features in common, and for this reason so do textbooks on both subjects. Any 'Champion's way to a lower handicap' invariably starts with the elements of technique, which in themselves are pure and untouched by failure. The master then takes the reader blow by blow through his successful defence of a major event at Pebble Beach or Augusta, showing how the ideal stroke sometimes achieves perfection and sometimes does not. It is emphasized that the art at this point is not to collapse at the cruelties of fate, but to achieve perfection by a different route; to rein in emotion, concentrate on one manoeuvre at a time and not be afraid of the possible implications on the final outcome. Retinal surgery calls for precisely these qualities.

The aim of this surgery is to achieve a flat, functioning retina at the first operation. The first attempt should be the best, but may, alas, not be the only one. A simple retinal detachment is one that is not yet complicated. Macular malfunction, retinal shrinkage and vitreal or anterior chamber haemorrhage can all turn the simplest of detachments into a nightmare. The patient must be forewarned of these possibilities in the most optimistic way, and this is the first surgical step. Thereafter, the remaining steps are:
1. To find the break(s)
2. To seal the break(s)
3. To prevent the break(s) from reopening.

Many methods are available to achieve these aims, but all must do so without compromising the flow of blood through the central retinal artery.

At our disposal are the following:
1. The binocular indirect ophthalmoscope and scleral depression, to discover the breaks
2. Cryopexy or laser, to induce the appropriate inflammation around the break(s)

**Figure 6.1**
Adhesion alone may not be enough. Cryopexy may increase the tractional force, and a scleral buckle reduces the risk that the break might reopen.

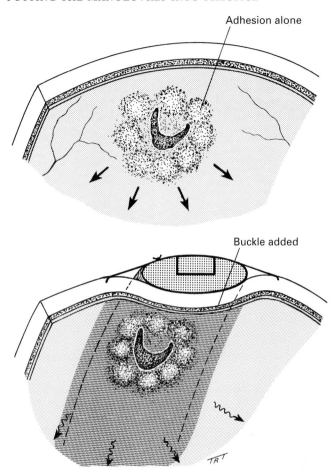

3. Air/gas in the vitreal cavity, to seal the break(s) from within

4. An encircling silicone band, which counters traction generally and provides a way of both holding a guttered explant in position and of allowing it to be moved, should the first position chosen prove to be wrong

5. Explants of various sorts (sponges, solid silicone rubber), the deployment of which will be influenced by the nature of the break(s)

6. Paracentesis, to make space for manoeuvres and to preserve the integrity of the central retinal artery

7. Release of subretinal fluid, to:
   (a) allow accurate cryopexy and buckling
   (b) allow a dialysis to settle on the inflammatory reaction
   (c) make space within the eye to allow necessary manoeuvres without closing the central retinal artery.

Some retinal detachments may call for only a selection of these manoeuvres, others may need all of them. The art is to progress as though moving along a wide boulevard, occasionally making a detour to one side or the other, but constantly driving forward and retracing our steps only when the eye dictates.

## MYOPIA

Most myopic detachments arise from a horseshoe break on the equator. Although the size of the balloons may appear dominant, the only important factor is the depth of subretinal fluid in the area of the break. The balloons may look fearsome, but they have no influence on the surgery, and the subretinal fluid should not be released just because it is there.

Preoperative flattening of the retina with bed rest is beneficial in two ways; first, it may reduce the complexity of subsequent surgery, and secondly, it encourages the retina to settle. Detachments that refuse to settle forewarn that the surgical plan may call for more rather than less.

**Figure 6.2**
A detachment is as shallow as the depth of the fluid under the break. Further shallowing with bed rest prior to surgery indicates the likelihood of successful flattening with minimal intervention.

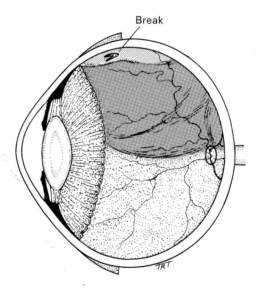

Break

The next step is to determine whether the break will settle on the indent produced by a scleral explant, without fluid release. If this can be achieved, without closing the central retinal artery, the operation is complete. If not, the following procedure should be followed:

1. If the central retinal artery is threatened, then the intraocular pressure may be reduced by repeated paracentesis, the first in anticipation of such an event before the buckle is applied.
2. Should the break not seem to settle happily on the buckle, then internal sealing with intravitreal air may be consid-

**Figure 6.3**
(1) Contiguous cryopexy around the break; (2) break placed on anterior slope of the buckle; (3) the buckle may be moved without additional weightbearing sutures, from one contour line to another or from one meridian to another.

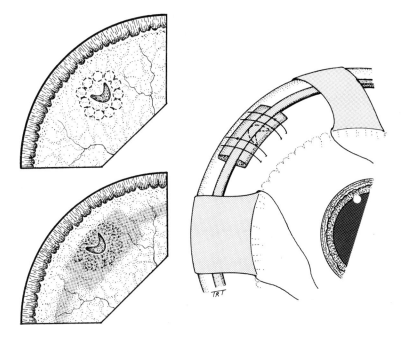

ered if the eye is soft enough to allow this without causing subsequent closure of the central retinal artery.

3. If at this point the break still remains defiantly open, then (and only then) might we consider the release of subretinal fluid to make space for the new manoeuvre. **NB:** Subretinal fluid cannot be released before the intraocular pressure is allowed to return to normal by releasing the tension sutures.

4. If the operation has not succeeded so far, for the reasons described, then enough fluid may remain under the tear to allow fluid release at this point. The avascularity of the underlying choroid must determine the exact site, which must be located with great accuracy. The collapsing effect

**Figure 6.4**
The classic retinal break of intracapsular extraction. This may still be found after cataract extraction complicated by vitreous loss, and after Yag capsulotomy.

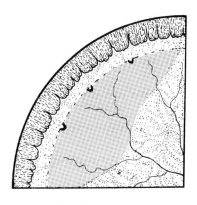
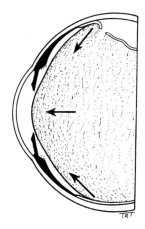

of a copious flow on the globe can be countered with preplaced weightbearing sutures, a bubble of air into the vitreous, or both.

5. All these manoeuvres presuppose that the surgeon has searched the contour line bearing the break to ensure that other unsuspected breaks do not threaten elsewhere in the retina. The clue to any such breaks is frequently found in the vitreous, in the form of wisps of operculated retina. Retinal disease around the same contour line might be contained more safely by an encircling band. If the balloons of fluid prevent the location of such breaks with certainty, then of course the fluid must be released and the ocular volume and pressure made up with the tension buckle and air as before.

## THE RIGID RETINA

Preretinal traction is unmistakable. The disease process puckers the retinal surface into star folds, pulls open multiple tears and rolls their edges. Retina and vitreous both move with a dull inertia, and rapidly come to a halt after one or two oscillations.

**Figure 6.5**
A rigid retina, with traction on the operculum, star folds, an immobile vitreous and multiple breaks on different contour lines. Conventional surgery is unlikely to succeed, and techniques used include vitrectomy, released traction, gas:air/fluid exchange, cryopexy or laser and reduction of intraocular volume.

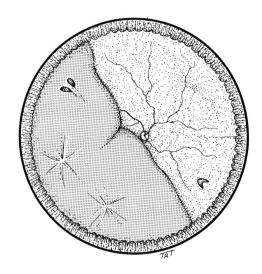

The same principles of surgery apply, but because higher buckles are indicated, space must be made to protect the central retinal artery. This can only be achieved by release of subretinal fluid. Good surgery (like good golf) rolls three shots into two, and a further benefit of fluid release is that it allows the retina to settle on the frozen chorioretinal bed – and hopefully to stay there.

If the buckles have not taken up the spare ocular volume, this can be made up with an injection of air into the vitreal cavity. This air bubble does not have to be used specifically to catch all the tears on its summit in the postoperative period, and there is no need to inflict immobility on the patient. Such calls for immobility belong to the early days of retinal surgery, and effective closure of the break(s) makes this unnecessary in most cases.

Whether an air bubble has been used or not, the patient should leave the theatre with the major break uppermost so that gravity will disperse potential subretinal fluid from the adhering edges of the break. If the retina is in contact with the buckle, then early mobilization the following day will not make it redetach. The 'break upwards' position is doubly indicated if air has been used because a bubble floats upwards, and it would be waste of this useful quality if the patient was not positioned with the break lying on the summit of the bubble.

The management of lower quadrant breaks hardly differs at all from that of upper quadrant breaks, except that dependence on an air bubble may call for an uncomfortable postoperative position with the face down into the pillow, head down, or both. Twenty-four hours in this position may be enough; once the tear is dry on the buckle then it is unlikely to open again unless under the influence of traction.

### The six-week recurrence

There is one particular instance where a rigid retina can be diagnosed with confidence despite the lack of its well-known associates such as a severe uveitis or intravitreal haemorrhage. This particular detachment presents initially with multiple tears occupying different contour lines, anywhere from the ora serrata to well behind the equator. Although their sizes may vary, they all share the horseshoe shape due to abnormal vitreoretinal adhesion. The taut opercula, the curled edges and the visible vitreal strands leave no doubt that traction is the main element.

The problem is that such retinae respond very well to conventional surgery in the first instance. The vitreal cutter contributes by revealing obvious tractional strands and making space for a bubble of $SF_6$, and all goes well for about 40 days. The tears then pull open, leaving gaping holes and a retina of increasing rigidity.

In the presence of such gaping breaks, silicone oil would almost certainly end up on the deep surface of the retina as well as in the vitreal cavity. If silicone oil is to be used the tears must be buckled first, and if they lie behind the equator such closure may not be possible. However, heavy liquid introduced in front of the optic nerve head can fill the vitreal cavity from the posterior pole forwards, clearing subretinal fluid through the retinal breaks and, by flattening the retina, reducing the temptation for the heavy liquid to pass through into the subretinal space.

Once the retina is flat, widespread laser photocoagulation may hold it in place.

The behaviour of detachments with such multiple tears is so predictable that bypassing the conventional buckle may well give the retina a better chance of flattening and of remaining flat.

## APHAKIA

Some 4% of patients went on to develop detachment of the retina following intracapsular cataract extraction. With the increasing popularity of the extracapsular method, this figure has been reduced to 0.5%.

Even in the absence of actual loss, the forward movement of the vitreous pulls on the vitreal base and in doing so pulls open little tears, which commonly lie just behind the ora serrata. Because traction is to blame the tears are frequently multiple, and because they are so peripheral they take on the colour of the choroid deep to them – which is anything but red. They are so small that even that nondescript choroidal appearance may not be noticed, and the clue to their presence lies in the little tags of retina seen wisping on the horizon.

The vitreal base itself is recognized as a line lying parallel to and behind the ora serrata. It should not be forgotten that the incidence of detachment produced by extracapsular

**Figure 6.6**
A 'goat's beard' of retina flung into profile by the scleral depressor.

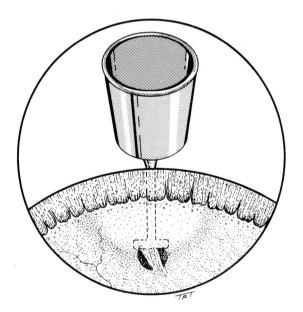

extraction rises to the former level of 4% when the Yag laser has violated the posterior cavity of the eye. At this point the surgeon may wish that the cataract had been removed in the old way, because capsular debris, lens implants and, worse still, pupil-fixated lens implants all conspire to obscure the critical area of the retina from the surgeon.

**Figure 6.7**
The vitreal base straddles the ora serrata. Classic breaks are to be found in its posterior border following cataract extraction complicated by vitreous loss or Yag capsulotomy.

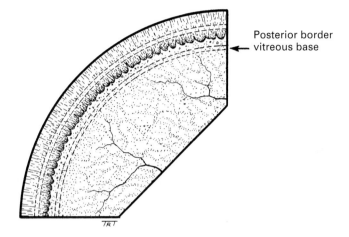

Posterior border
← vitreous base

The technique:

1. The area bearing the break, by virtue of its close proximity to the anterior attachment of the retina at the ora serrata, is frequently shallow. For this reason, simple buckling with a guttered explant held in place by an encircling silicone band may be sufficient.

2. Necessary space for manoeuvre can be created by paracentesis, even after an intracapsular extraction. It is however important that formed vitreous is not released through the corneal opening in place of aqueous, because that will compound the pathology that brought the patient to the retinal surgeon in the first place.

3. A gaping break can be sealed onto the buckle by an air bubble, if space allows. Unfortunately the bubble may also steal forwards into the anterior chamber, where it will separate into several small bubbles. Injection should therefore be delayed until we are absolutely certain that we do not want to look at the fundus again in detail.

4. If the tear continues to stand off the buckle and gives any hint of rigidity in doing so, then release of subretinal fluid is the only useful way of bringing the layers into contact.

5. Aphakic detachments (which are not infrequently rigid) call for a slightly tighter band than normal, and possibly a slightly higher buckle. Given these special requirements, subretinal fluid release may be indicated more often than if the detachment is shallow and mobile.

6. Should the breaks (unusually) dominate in the lower quadrants of the eye, then accurate buckling at the time of surgery should be depended upon rather than an air bubble.

Aphakia does not necessarily mean that the detachment itself is aphakic. It may well be a myopic detachment in someone who just happens to have had a cataract removed. In these circumstances, the equator is the contour at risk because of the myopia, but the retro-oral contour should be suspect also because of the aphakia (See Figures 4.6 and 4.7). **NB:** Both contours may be affected.

## DIALYSIS

Congenital weakness in the retina may give rise to a crack just behind the ora serrata, and these cracks are often found in the lower temporal quadrants of both eyes, although one may be considerably more advanced than in the other. The presence of a tide mark or multiple tide marks guides us to the source of the subretinal fluid.

The technique:

1. Cryopexy must be applied where the retina is going to settle into place, and we often find that this is never exactly at the ora but rather further back than we might have imagined. Cryopexy should therefore be applied in a continual line, starting at the ora serrata in healthy retina and continuing behind the edge of the dialysis into healthy retina beside the ora serrata at the other extremity.

**Figure 6.8**
Dialysis. Unless the retina is very rigid, most cases of dialysis will settle on a plain circumferential explant. The technique includes cryopexy (where the retina will settle, not where it is lying at the outset), release of subretinal fluid (which is always thick) and buckling (not always right up to the rectus insertions).
Continued gaping may be closed by a fragment of silastic sponge deep to the explant.

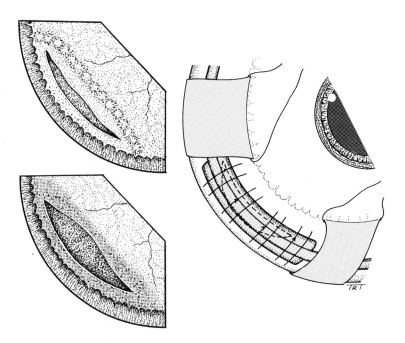

2. In cases of dialysis, subretinal fluid must always be released because simple buckling (although tempting) always results in a procession of all the retinal layers towards the centre, with the vital layers defiantly separated by the thick subretinal fluid.
3. If copious subretinal fluid is released, then we must anticipate sudden collapse of intraocular volume by having the tension sutures preplaced for rapid tying. Sometimes even that is not enough, and an air bubble can make up the rest.
4. A rigid retina again calls for a slightly tighter band and a slightly higher buckle, and whatever the state of the retina, it is of course useful to check the other eye whilst the patient is in theatre and under anaesthetic.

Postoperative care follows that of other detachments. If, however, air has been injected, it is as well to use it. The patient may therefore spend the first postoperative night with the head tilted slightly downwards and the dialysis as near to the summit of the air bubble as comfort will allow.

## DISINSERTION

Unlike a dialysis, where a frill of retina remains attached behind the ora serrata, a disinsertion is traumatic avulsion of the ora serrata itself. Damage frequently extends beyond the retina–vitreal haemorrhage and rising intraocular pressure will remind us of the violent cause.

Management is identical to that of a dialysis, except that blood and the disruption of natural barriers within the eye must lead us to assume the greater possibility of preretinal retraction later – an assumption that is not always borne out. However, a slightly tighter than normal band and a slightly higher than normal buckle, even if not strictly necessary, cannot be too high a price to pay to ensure that the retina will not redetach.

Despite the history of injury, we must still look at the other eye. This is because the injury may have simply provoked a detachment in a vulnerable retina, in which case the fellow eye may harbour mirror image degeneration.

Postoperative management calls for nothing out of the ordinary, but the possibility of raised pressure after surgery is particularly likely if it was already elevated to begin with.

## OTHER TRAUMATIC BREAKS

In eyes bearing other evidence of trauma, often in the form of vitreal haemorrhage, retinal tears will by their very nature be of random distribution.

The technique:

1. Because the tears are ragged, they are more likely to unfold over an air bubble
2. Because of the haemorrhage and the ever-present possibility of preretinal retraction, the buckle and band should be both higher and tighter than normal
3. In order to make sufficient space for manoeuvre, there is usually no alternative but to release subretinal fluid
4. Such cases are better treated with vitrectomy, to remove clouds of vitreal debris and blood and to make space.

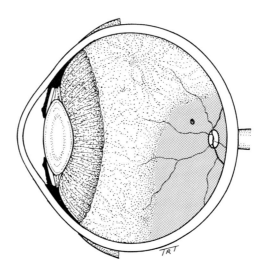

**Figure 6.9**
Failure of the subretinal fluid to reach the ora serrata always raises the possibility of a posterior polar break. Treatment includes vitrectomy (to make space), air/fluid exchange, air:gas/air exchange, platelets to macular hole, and cryopexy or laser to other retinal breaks.

## GIANT BREAK

In most retinal detachments, the surface area of the break is so small compared to that of the rest of the retina that it does not interfere in any way with the surgical replacement of the retina in its natural position. However, when the extent of a break reaches a critical point, its size can prevent the retina from being repositioned as it should. The surgical goals remain as before:

1. Find the break
2. Seal the break
3. Make the seal permanent and watertight.

To this is now added a fourth goal – to persuade the edges of the retinal break to return (as near as possible) to their original sites.

When a break (particularly one near the ora) extends farther than a quadrant, we move into the realms of a giant tear, which presents yet another surgical dilemma. Such breaks develop as they do because of a peculiar vitreoretinal abnormality which is almost certainly also present in the asymptomatic fellow eye.

Giant breaks are, in effect, giant dialyses, with a frill of retina persisting behind the ora serrata and a posterior flap which may obscure the optic nerve, dragged there by the persistent vitreoretinal adhesions which tore the retina in the first place.

To replace the retina where it belongs, the flap be unfolded and remain so.

### Release
A pars plana vitrectomy will cut and remove the abnormal vitreoretinal adhesions from the posterior flap and also make space for manoeuvre. As with all elegant surgery, two aims are achieved with one stroke.

### Unfolding
Many stratagems have been – and indeed still are – employed for unfolding the retina. These include the use of an air bubble, silicone oil, or heavy liquid. Perhaps the most successful method to date has been the use of heavy liquid (perfluorocarbon).

When vitrectomy is complete, the heavy liquid is injected as a bubble of increasing size over the optic nerve head and fills the vitreal cavity, picking up the retinal edge as it enlarges.

### Inflammatory reaction
The choice lies between external cryopexy or endolaser – the latter is possibly less likely to provoke vitreoretinal proliferation.

### Scleral buckle
Supporting the retinal edges on a gentle indent probably helps counter any residual tendency for the break to pull open again.

At this point, controversy sets in. The heavy liquid cannot be left in the eye indefinitely because of its feared toxicity, which is probably due to mechanical pressure rather than pharmacological causes. If the retina is in a good position, there is much to be said for leaving the heavy liquid until the inflammatory seal has become permanent – about four weeks. At this stage, an exchange of air for heavy liquid clears the eye of the offending material, and allows further tamponade with intravitreal air/gas.

There is, however, a sizeable group of vitreoretinal surgeons who oppose this two-stage approach because it involves a second invasion of the vitreal cavity. They prefer to carry out an air/heavy liquid exchange at the first operation, adding 20% $SF_6$, and using the tamponade of the air/gas mixture to produce a permanent seal.

# PNEUMATIC RETINOPEXY

The desire to simplify management and to treat a frank retinal detachment without open surgery led Hilton and Grizzard (1986) to consider the treatment of upper retinal detachments related to single or adjacent breaks with adhesion and gas tamponade.

There is no departure from the basic principles of:
1. Finding the break
2. Sealing the break
3. Making the seal watertight and permanent
4. Above all, creating space in the eye to allow whatever stratagem the eye might demand without simultaneous closure of the central retinal artery.

It is customary to apply intensive topical antibiotics for up to 24 hours before surgery. There is no hard rule about where the procedure should be carried out, but we must remember that we are violating the posterior cavity and asepsis, as for any standard procedure, is preferable.

### Anaesthesia
A combination of topical benoxinate and subconjunctival infiltration with 2% lignocaine (as for transconjunctival cryopexy) in the appropriate areas permits the necessary manipulation.

Controversy exists even at this point and some surgeons prefer a retrobulbar injection of anaesthesia.

### Making space
The intraocular pressure can be reduced by:
1. 250 mg of oral acetazolamide one hour before surgery
2. The application of a Honan bulb (as for cataract extraction)
3. Paracentesis
4. Cryopexy or laser (if the former is favoured, this will incidentally soften the eye further).

### The primary seal
Closure of the break(s) by flotation and surface tension is brought about by an intravitreal injection of pure $SF_6$, which doubles in size over the next eighteen hours. $C_3F_8$ takes longer (about 24 hours) to triple in size, and remains in place for longer.

### Technique
A rectus insertion (180 degrees from the breaks) is seized with the fixation forceps, and anterior to this must lie the pars plana. 0.4 ml $SF_6$ or 0.3 ml $C_3F_8$ is delivered precisely from a 1 ml syringe attached to a 25 or 30 gauge needle. The

5/8 needle is driven into the eye away from the lens, and the appropriate volumes of gas delivered into the vitreal cavity – a single movement of the plunger creating a single bubble. In our experience, the tuberculin syringe needle originally recommended is too flexible.

With that unchanging adherence to principles that should mark retinal surgery, the first object of our attention must be the optic nerve head, pallor of which indicates induced ischaemia. Secondly, note the central retinal artery, pulsation of which indicates that any more gas would be too much. Frank closure indicates a surfeit, and demands instant attention.

### Closure of the central retinal artery

Releasing gas is perfect in theory, and almost unachievable in practice. Tapping the paracentesis site should, however, release enough aqueous to restore pulsation.

### Postoperative management

The positioning of the break on the summit of the bubble must be explained to the patient, who may go home in about an hour following further measurement of the intraocular pressure and examination of the central retinal artery.

### The permanent inflammatory seal

Transconjunctival cryopexy, monitored through the binocular indirect ophthalmoscope, can be applied if the detachment is shallow enough for accurate placement. It brings with it two advantages:
1. It softens the eye further
2. The entire operation is completed on the same day.

Laser photocoagulation is best delivered through the binocular indirect ophthalmoscope, and brings its own advantages:
1. Evidence suggests that it is less likely to induce surface proliferation
2. If the retina has not flattened, then the door is left open for a conventional buckle with cryopexy being deployed at the time of surgery, and not 24–48 hours later.

## REFERENCES AND FURTHER READING

Alexandridis, E. and Kohl-Eisenhut, H. (1986). Treatment of retinal detachment with macular hole. *Graefe's Arch. Clin. Exp. Ophthalmol.*, **224**, 11–12.

Billington, B. M. and Leaver, P. K. (1986). Vitrectomy and fluid/silicone oil exchange for giant retinal tears: results at 18 months. *Graefe's Arch. Clin. Exp. Ophthalmol.*, **224**, 7–10.

Hilton, G. F. and Grizzard, W. S. (1986) Pneumatic retinopexy. A two step outpatient operation without conjunctival incision. *Ophthalmology*, **93**, 626.

# 7

# Vitrectomy

Posterior vitrectomy must rank with lens implantation as one of the greatest advances in ophthalmic surgery in the last fifty years. However, in common with so many significant innovations, it requires the rejection of the accepted wisdom of a hundred years. Generations of eye surgeons have looked upon the loss of formed vitreous as a mortal sin, to be followed relentlessly by aphakic retinal detachment, aphakic glaucoma, and what is now known as macular oedema, or by anxiety about all three.

Conventional treatment called for rapid wound closure, leaving the pupil dragged up to the suture line by a sheet of vitreous, like a hammock. Such an approach was founded on the assumption that if the loss of vitreous was bad, then the loss of less vitreous would be better. It took Thorpe in 1963 and Kasner in 1969 to demonstrate that whilst the loss of vitreous in itself is of course important, *how it is lost* is infinitely more important. Kasner's response to loss was to lose more, but in a controlled fashion – absorbing the gel on surgical spears and carefully minimizing traction with the painstaking section of the vitreal strands. In due course the vitreous fell back behind a concave iris, and no strands distorted the roundness of the pupil or threatened the integrity of the corneoscleral wound. From such brilliant simplicity was anterior vitrectomy born.

Initial attempts to take this technique into the posterior cavity through a widened corneoscleral wound – the so called 'open sky' technique – soon gave way to the closed approach through the pars plana.

In 1971 Machemer described his vitreous infusion suction cutter, and from these equally brilliant inspirations the range of surgical options we now take for granted has been developed.

There are specific indications for vitrectomy in relation to retinal detachment:
1. If vitreal opacities – either blood or debris – prevent the conventional management of a retinal detachment
2. If space within the eye cannot be made by conventional means, such as subretinal fluid release or paracentesis, or

when a posterior polar detachment does not spread far
enough forwards to allow for safe subretinal fluid release
3. When some pathological process threatens the vitreal cavity within and prevents visualization from without
4. When direct manipulation of some intraocular tissue is
required
5. When vitreal adhesion tears a quadrant or more of retina
from an intact ora serrata and its attached frill of peripheral retina.

## ESSENTIAL PRINCIPLES

A probe combining the capabilities of section and suction is
introduced through the pars plana into the vitreal cavity.

Abstraction of intravitreal contents will lead to total collapse of the globe unless its volume is maintained by an in-
flow (also through the pars plana) of some compatible fluid,
such as Ringer's lactate.

Illumination is provided by a light probe through another
quadrant of the pars plana or, in certain circumstances, by the
binocular indirect ophthalmoscope.

## TECHNIQUE

The conjunctiva is opened around the limbus, as for a retinal
detachment. Any surface vessels on the sclera over the pars
plana on the upper temporal and lower temporal meridians
are cauterized. A point anterior to the rectus insertions (and,
hence, the ora serrata) but sufficiently posterior to the limbus
to protect the lens is selected for the in-flow.

A mattress suture of 5/0 polyester or polyglactin is preplaced in the sclera over the temporal pars plana, just below
the horizontal meridian. An MVR blade – shaped like a
miniature spear – is passed between the limbs of the suture,
its flat surface parallel to the limbus. The in-flow, free of
bubbles, is passed through this opening, and the loop of the
stay suture is secured over the plate of the in-flow cannula.
The free ends are then knotted over the other end of the plate.
Positioning the cannula without stripping the ciliary epithelium and without excessive angulation is often the hardest
part of the whole operation. If the in-flow is securely in the
vitreal cavity, pressure on the globe of the cannula will be
seen to produce movement of random bubbles of air in the
tubing. Two further openings are then made in the same way,
using the MVR blade, through the temporal and nasal pars

**Figure 7.1**
Set up for vitrectomy. All
sclerotomies are anterior to the rectus
muscles, and the in-flow plate is held
flat whilst the sutures are tied.

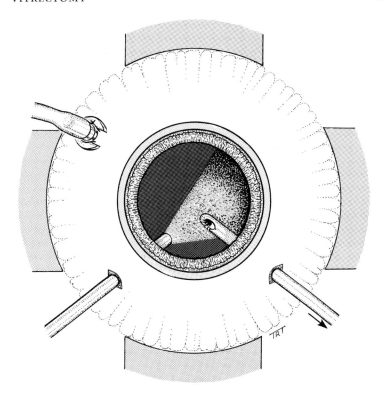

plana just above the three and nine o'clock meridians. The
stage is now set for vitrectomy.

### Illumination

A 19-gauge probe, connected to a light source by a fibreoptic
cable, enters the vitreal cavity through the upper nasal stab
incision.

### Visualization

A plano-concave corneal contact lens allows the surgeon to
focus the operating microscope onto any level of the vitreal
cavity. There are many such lenses. One requires the luxury
of an assistant who does nothing other than hold it in position on the cornea, whilst others can be fixed by a ring
sutured to the sclera. Others still are self-retaining, and float
on a film of sodium hyaluronate.

It is also possible, and indeed desirable in certain circumstances, to visualize the entire procedure through the binocular indirect ophthalmoscope – in this case a light probe would
be superfluous.

### The suction cutter

Different machines have different settings, but the essential basic
requirement is to have suction reduced to the lowest level compatible with adequate removal of vitreal contents. Instruments

**Figure 7.2**
Clearing the midvitreal cavity and
incidentally making space. The port is
pointing away from the retina.

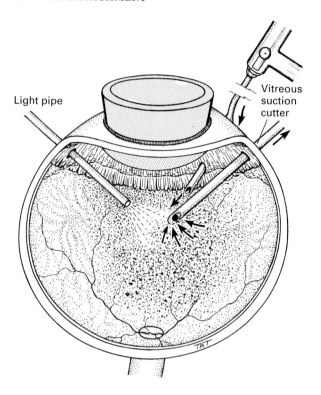

commonly used today tend to function at 150 mm/Hg. Anything stronger, although apparently tolerated by the eye during the operation, may inflict suction damage on the flat retina,
and this can reveal itself much later when breaks pull open in
the retina for no very obvious reason. The original cutters
employed an oscillating blade that could be modified in
speed, range and balance. However, experience over the years
has shown that a guillotine action at the highest frequency
possible offers the greatest safety to the eye, by laying emphasis on the section of intravitreal debris rather than on suction.

### After surgery

Once the vitrectomy has been completed, certain steps must
be followed. On the assumption that manipulation by the
fibreoptic and the suction cutter may have damaged the adjacent retina, it is customary to apply cryopexy to the adjacent
ora serrata in each of these sites, which should be examined
meticulously for possible breaks – either induced or inciden-
tal. Although there should be no movement around the in-
flow, some surgeons extend this cryopexy to involve the
lower temporal ora serrata as well.

The sclerotomies need to be sutured firmly, and failure to
do so may result in later collapse of the eye. Different surgeons recommend different suturing techniques and indeed
different sutures, but we have found that 7/0 polyglactin

**Figure 7.3**
Plugs are used to block the
sclerotomies when not in use.

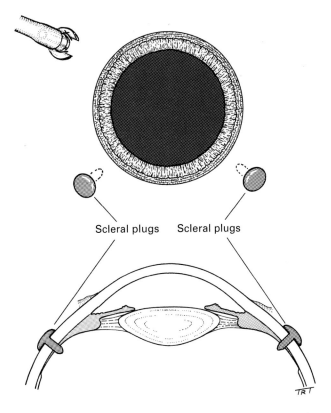

**Figure 7.3**
Plugs are used to block the
sclerotomies when not in use.

Scleral plugs    Scleral plugs

combines ease of use with strength. Squeezing the in-flow, or
turning it off at the three-way tap, allows the sutures to be
tied against no resistance.

It is critical not to put any pressure on the eye after the in-
flow has been removed, for fear of producing hypotony by
needless expression of the now liquid intravitreal contents. A
preplaced bow knot is perhaps the best way to prevent this.

In all circumstances, the needle should be inserted into the
sclera away from the retina to avoid the addition of a needless retinal break to the existing pathology.

## THE ESSENTIAL MANOEUVRES

As with conventional retinal surgery, vitrectomy is made up
of a series of legitimate manoeuvres. All are available for use,
but may not necessarily be used in the same order or indeed
every time.

### Binocular indirect ophthalmoscope

The reduced magnification using this instrument is trivial
compared to the extended field of view during certain manoeuvres such as endodiathermy, endolaser photocoagulation,

internal drainage of subretinal fluid and air/fluid/gas/silicone oil/heavy liquid exchanges. Mastering the technique teaches other skills needed in vitreoretinal surgery, and small-diameter lenses permit an almost coaxial view of the lower nasal quadrants.

### Flute needle

This has a handle with a single finger stop hole (whence its name) connecting to a blunt-tipped 19-gauge cannula, and is an essential and simple device upon which many of the fundamental actions of vitrectomy depend. It is in effect an intraocular vacuum cleaner, the power coming from the fluid inflow which drives the vacuum whilst the finger stop controls the vacuum with great precision.

Under direct observation, the flute needle may be taken down to the surface of the retina to remove blood. It may also be inserted through a retinal tear to the deep surface of the retina, to drain subretinal fluid internally. It plays a vital part in the exchanges that take place within the vitreal cavity between Ringer's lactate, silicone oil, air, gas and heavy liquid.

In more sophisticated versions, it is possible to reverse the flow (for example, to free retina trapped in the tip).

### Air exchange

A completed vitrectomy leaves the vitreal cavity full of Ringer's lactate solution, which of course has no surface tension effect on the retinal break. Air however does have this effect, and can be delivered to the eye from an automated air machine kept at a constant pressure. The exact pressure must

**Figure 7.4**
Air/fluid exchange. Air drives the fluid out through the flute needle, and will eventually fill the vitreal cavity.

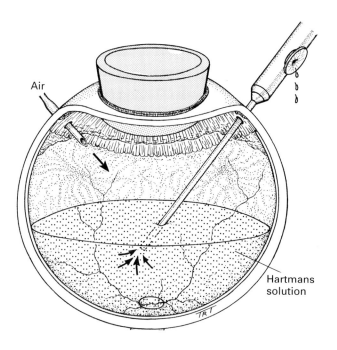

Air

Hartmans
solution

be chosen by the surgeon, but 40 mm/Hg seems to offer a pressure level that facilitates scleral manoeuvres without threat to the central retinal artery. The automated device drives air into the vitreal cavity through the three-way tap on the inflow, and Ringer's lactate out of the vitreal cavity through the flute needle. The fluid level around the cannula can easily be seen falling back to the retinal surface, and as the needle tip becomes free of the Ringer's lactate solution, the fluid flowing from the finger hole begins to froth. This action can be predicted by watching the fluid level clinging to the flute needle decrease as it gives way to air.

In aphakic eyes the view is sometimes lost to begin with, and selecting the best position for the flute needle before inserting the air prevents the view from being lost at a critical juncture. When the manoeuvre is complete, the sclerotomies should be closed as described above. If air alone is not enough, then a 20% mixture of $SF_6$ (one part gas to four parts air) is drawn into a 20 ml syringe and injected into the vitreal cavity via the three-way tap, whilst the 'pure air' escapes up the flute needle.

It cannot be emphasized enough that faulty closure of sclerotomies can lead to extreme hypotony and large choroidal effusions, and we can end up with worse problems than before the surgery.

### Internal drainage
Conventional subretinal fluid release is not without its complications – choroidal haemorrhage, incarceration and hypotony, to name but three.

**Figure 7.5**
Internal drainage and air/fluid exchange. The retina is perforated with sharp point diathermy and the air in-flow drives the subretinal fluid out through the flute needle.

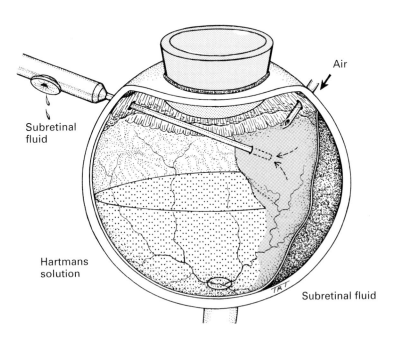

Subretinal fluid

Air

Hartmans solution

Subretinal fluid

If the existing retinal break is easily accessible, then sub-retinal fluid can be directed up the flute needle directly through the break. Proper finger closure at the point of passage into the subretinal space prevents the retina from being driven into the tube as well. Flattening of the retina can be magically swift.

Occasionally subretinal fluid cannot be drained through an existing break. In such circumstances it is still possible – and indeed safer – to drain internally, creating a retinal hole in a position of our choosing. An endodiathermy 'sharp point' seals off any potential bleeding as it makes the necessary perforation through which the subretinal fluid may be drained.

## Endodiathermy

Intraocular bipolar diathermy can be delivered in two ways:
1. A single probe with two electrodes separated by insulation is ideal for producing drainage retinotomies and (in its flat-tipped version) for coagulating surface bleeding spots.
2. The diathermy leads can also be attached to the light probe and whatever instrument is passing through the other upper sclerotomy. Using these instruments within the eye is a more effective way of achieving haemostasis from elevated sources of bleeding.

Any bleeding vessels can be cauterized **EXCEPT** for those sprouting directly from the optic nerve head. Diathermy applied to these will certainly destroy them, but will also destroy the optic nerve, completely negating any value derived from a blood-free vitreal cavity.

The strength of endodiathermy delivered varies with different machines. It is a useful tip to check that the tips are working and to test their strength by observing their effect on surface scleral vessels.

## Endolaser

Various lasers are now available, with wavelengths ranging from argon green through the solid state equivalents and on to diode in the infrared waveband. The power is transmitted along a fibreoptic cable, which (like all fibreoptic cables) cannot function if sharply angulated. The operator and assistants must be protected with an appropriate filter incorporated in the microscope or with goggles when using the binocular indirect ophthalmoscope. The patient is equally vulnerable, and it must be remembered that delivery *within* the eye calls for reduced power settings because the light is not required to negotiate the cornea, lens and anterior vitreous before landing on the retina.

The spot size decreases as the probe approaches the retina, and the intensity increases as the probe approaches the retina. As with all forms of laser application, treatment is possible only if the retina is flat.

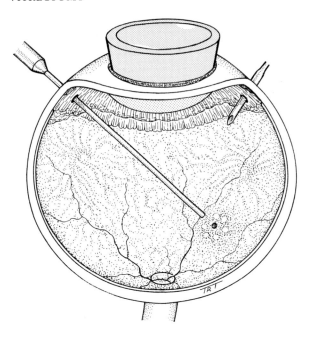

## Silicone oil (polydimethyl-siloxane)

Anyone faced with large numbers of retinal detachments must find cases where the closure of breaks is defeated by preretinal traction, which pulls them open again despite a high buckle. In such cases, the solution to the problem may be intravitreal silicone oil. This will physically hold the retina physically in position, provided:

1. The surface membranes are removed
2. The vitreal cavity is completely filled with silicone oil
3. The entrance to the break is closed with a buckle. Silicone oil has limited surface tension, unlike air, and will readily pass through the larger break into the subretinal space

Silicone oil is lighter than water, and for this reason the vitreal cavity must first be filled with air, which is lighter still. This can therefore be displaced from below upwards as the oil falls into the deepest part of the vitreal cavity.

After the air/ fluid exchange (using the ubiquitous flute needle), the same manoeuvre is applied to the silicone oil with the air now escaping up the flute in place of Ringer's lactate. Because of its high viscosity, the oil is forced into the in-flow under pressure at the three-way tap. This demands heavy-duty tubing and connections, otherwise the system will discharge the oil uselessly on to the scleral surface, the surgeon's glove and every essential instrument.

Many vitrectomy units today have a silicone pump, but a simple syringe, firmly held, serves equally well.

It is easy to replace all the air with silicone oil, but if the transfer is delayed unduly aqueous will begin to displace the

**Figure 7.7**
Injection of silicone oil must follow
air/fluid exchange. Care must be
taken not to over-inject, and
preplaced sutures must be ready to
close the sclerotomy. Biometry must
come before silicone infusion. It is
impossible afterwards.

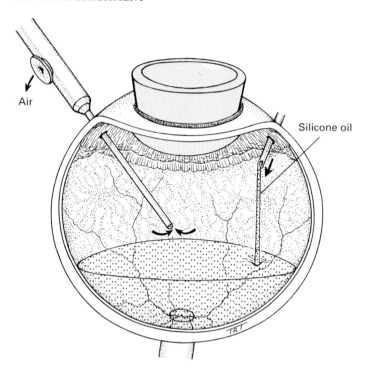

air, and silicone oil will definitely not be able to displace the
heavier aqueous. It is also easy to lose oil from the vitreal
cavity when the in-flow is removed and at the end of the procedure. A strong preplaced suture, tied immediately keeps the
oil where its presence was intended.

It is equally easy to close the central retinal artery, but just
as easy to avoid it if we realize that the intraocular pressure
can silently rise to dangerous levels.

Silicone oil is clearly not without its dangers:
1. It always results in a posterior subcapsular cataract
2. It can give rise to an intractable intraocular pressure rise
3. It can become emulsified and opaque
4. It can produce band degeneration and corneal opacifica-
   tion.

Oil with a high molecular weight and low polydispersion is
less prone to emulsification.

### Pseudophakia and silicone oil

The inevitable cataract eventually calls for extraction, and
lens implantation calls for biometry. The inaccuracy of such
measurements in these circumstances, however, makes biometry valueless. The axial length cannot be measured accurately
because detached retina effectively shortens the axial length,
and a vitreal cavity full of silicone will not allow biometry.

A peripheral iridectomy at six o'clock reduces the risk of
oil-induced pupil block.

Silicone oil cannot be used in pseudophakic patients whose intraocular lens is also made of silicone.

### To remove or not to remove

There is some controversy about what to do with the oil once it is in position. Removing it avoids the above two complications, but may well result in the relapse of the original detachment. It is our experience that the patient's well-being is best served by leaving the oil in position, and dealing with the complications if and when they occur. For such prolonged tamponade, oil of a higher viscosity (such as 5700 centistokes) is preferred. Lower viscosity oil (1300 centistokes) is more easily injected and more easily removed, if removal is the preferred technique.

### Removal

If the oil has to go, then exchange cannot take place with a flute needle. Even 1300 centistoke oil is too viscous to be removed in this way, and it must be driven out through an opening in the upper pars plana by an infusion line of Ringer's lactate.

### Heavy liquids (perfluorocarbons)

If silicone oil floats on aqueous, then aqueous floats on perfluorocarbon, and this can therefore replace aqueous from

**Figure 7.8**
Giant tear. Treatment includes vitrectomy and the removal of traction bands. Heavy liquid will flatten the retina from below, squeezing the subretinal fluid out through the giant break.

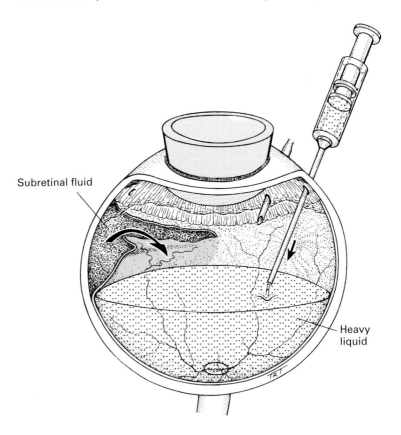

Subretinal fluid

Heavy liquid

below upwards. Liquids vary because of their side chains, but perfluorodecalin ($C_{10}F_{19}$) has many of the following desired qualities:

1. They should be colourless and optically clear
2. They have a high specific gravity and sink into the lower cavity of the eye; they are therefore useful for cases involving surface traction
3. They have a reasonable surface tension, somewhere between that of air and silicone oil, so that tears can be sealed
4. They must be inert
5. They produce a very definite interface with air or Ringer's lactate, allowing easy recognition of the bubble during surgery.

The fluid is introduced by direct injection over the optic nerve head using a syringe and a blunt-tipped cannula. The surgeon may choose to control the syringe by hand or by word of mouth to an assistant, in which case the cannula will be connected with silicone tubing to a safely remote syringe. As the intraocular pressure inevitably rises, the light probe is temporarily withdrawn to allow Ringer's lactate to escape.

During an exchange monitored with the indirect ophthalmoscope, the same intermittent control of pressure can be achieved by withdrawing the blunt cannula.

Some may argue that the heavy liquid should be replaced with air or air and gas at the end of the procedure, thus completing the operation in one stage. It must certainly be removed at some point, because although it is not chemically toxic to the retina, its weight in the long term is thought to be physically damaging to the retinal cells. Its presence in the anterior chamber is also known to be damaging to the corneal endothelium.

Heavy liquids were originally used to seal rigid lower breaks, when their weight could flatten the retina by pushing the subretinal fluid through the break into the vitreal cavity. Because it fills the vitreal cavity against the retina, it can express fluid from the subretinal space in the presence of lower or multiple breaks. It can also unroll the edge of a giant retinal tear.

The flattening will not be permanent in any of these circumstances unless traction bands and membranes are removed.

Once the heavy liquid has achieved the flattening or unrolling, then sealing of the retinal break follows the usual sequence:

1. An appropriate chorioretinal inflammation, preferably applied with widespread laser rather than with cryopexy.
2. Scleral buckling – although, because there is a degree of surface tension, tight closure is not critical and nor is a complete fill necessary, except in the presence of multiple upper breaks which cannot benefit from a fluid favouring the lower quadrants of the globe.

**NB**: All of the above manoeuvres can of course be carried out with the microscope and an appropriate contact lens, and it is up to the surgeon which view is to be chosen.

The liquid is usually left long enough to allow firm adhesion to take place – about four weeks.

### Removal

Heavy liquid has to be withdrawn by suction whilst an infusion of Ringer's lactate solution maintains the ocular volume. A flute tip on a 20 ml syringe (for manual extraction) or the suction cutter (using suction alone) will draw a mixture of heavy liquid and infusion fluid from the centre of the vitreal cavity. Suction is continued in this way until the surfaces of the reducing bubble of heavy liquid are seen to take shape over the optic nerve head. At this point, the suction dips deeper and deeper into the bubble until no more heavy liquid remains.

## SPECIFIC INDICATIONS FOR VITRECTOMY

### Vitreal opacities

Surgery aims first to reveal what needs to be done. Obscuring blood or other opaque materials are removed, and their removal incidentally makes space for subsequent surgical manipulation. Surface membranes must be removed; such membranes pucker the retina like kitchen clingfilm, and unless they are removed, the retina will remain puckered and detached.

**Figure 7.9**
Right-angled intravitreal scissors cutting surface membranes.

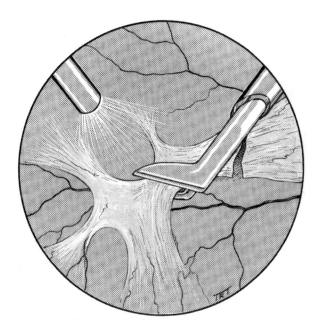

## Making space

If subretinal fluid release is not possible and a paracentesis insufficient, then vitreal removal is the safest alternative to preserve the patency of the central retinal artery if scleral buckling and air injection threaten it with closure.

## Giant retinal tear

There are two fundamental features of giant tears:
1. There is always gross vitreal pathology that has to be dealt with
2. The retinal break is too large to return naturally to its starting point.

### *Management*

1. Vitrectomy, to make space and cut the traction bands
2. Heavy liquid, to unroll the edges
3. Laser – if the retina is now flat – in three rows just behind the retinal edge
4. Encircling band. A guttered explant may not always be necessary, and indeed may prevent the retinal edge from settling
5. Air/fluid exchange
6. Air/$SF_6$(20%)/air exchange.

## Macular hole

Full depth perforation of the macula is rare, and is generally the result of:
1. Trauma
2. Myopia
3. An unknown cause – usually in postmenopausal women.

Gass first considered the pathogenesis of idiopathic senile macular holes in 1988 and graded them as follows:
1. Convexity over the fovea
2. Convexity plus perforation over the fovea
3. Full-thickness macular hole
4. Full-thickness macular hole plus complete vitreal detachment, sometimes together with partial elevation of the retina around the macula.

Surgery was carried out for this in the past, and in 1966 Rosengren described a technique involving a spherical macular buckle and intravitreal air. The advent of vitrectomy and intravitreal $SF_6$ or $C_3F_8$ has raised interest again in macular hole surgery.

The aims are:
1. To prevent the retina from detaching
2. To restore the macula to its normal position
3. To retain some degree of central visual function.

The technique involves vitrectomy (particularly removing any residual vitreous over the macula) and an intravitreal mixture of gas and air in routine concentration, followed by strict face down posturing for several days.

In place of the usual inflammatory reaction, a platelet extract from the patient's own blood may be placed around the edges of the macula.

The jury is still out on the efficacy of this surgery. Technically it is not difficult for the surgeon, but the face down posturing is difficult for the patient, particularly when extended over several days without any improvement in central vision to show for it. There is also the possibility of other complications.

### Retinotomy and retinectomy

The retina normally lines the concave posterior cavity from the disc to the ora serrata. Pathology of one form or another can result in retinal shortening, reducing its ability to take up a normal concave shape. In pre-vitrectomy days the only recourse was a high buckle, and indeed that may still be the most satisfactory answer.

The exact causes are unknown, but associated pathology includes:
1. Intraocular haemorrhage
2. Inflammation
3. Incarceration of the retina in the sclera, due to either trauma or surgery
4. Contraction of the retina, due to either simple fibrosis or proliferative retinopathy (PVR).

When a buckle is not adequate, then vitrectomy must be used to relieve traction and remove all tractional membranes. If these aims are carried out properly, the retina will usually be amenable to one of the surgical techniques already described. If however extensive shortening of the retina continues after membrane removal, then a relaxing cut in the retina may be considered, along the lines described by Machemer *et al.* (1986).

Prior to cutting the retina, heavy diathermy obliterates potential bleeding vessels. As with giant tears, perfluorocarbon may be used to persuade the posterior edge of the detachment to return to the near normal position. The remaining retina is now avascular and a possible source of cellular proliferation, therefore it is best excised.

Internal tamponade with air and gas, with or without a scleral buckle, may in certain cases allow the retina to fix permanently to the adhesion brought about by a triple row of laser photocoagulation scars.

### Endophthalmitis

Any invasion of the ocular cavity, whether by uncontrolled trauma or controlled surgery, carries with it the risk of invasion by micro-organisms. Should this occur, the patient will certainly complain of a dramatic increase in pain. However, a decrease in the level of vision is a harder symptom to evaluate, particularly if it was not very good to begin with. A painful eye that suddenly becomes diffusely red, giving cloudy vision for the patient and an equally cloudy view into the eye for the surgeon, presents unambiguously the dreaded calamity of intraocular infection.

Micro-organisms generally enter the eye via a penetrating ocular injury, but infection can appear (to the dismay of the surgeon) following what appeared to have been an uncomplicated intraocular operation. It can of course also overwhelm the defence mechanisms of the eye in patients who are immunologically compromised, either by systemic disease or by ongoing chemotherapy.

The first principle of treatment is to recognize that the unthinkable has happened, whilst the second is to find the offending organism and if possible destroy it with an appropriate antibiotic. The third, in parallel with the second, is to limit the damage wrought on the eye by the intraocular inflammation. Initially, a broad sweep of antibiotic cover is delivered either by drop medication or by subconjunctival or intravitreal injection.

### Antibiotics

Amikacin sulphate is an aminoglycocide, which is active against a broad spectrum of gram negative organisms, particularly pseudomonas. It also has some antigram positive activity.

Vancomycin is an amphoteric glycopeptide, which is bactericidal against a broad range of gram positive organisms.

Ceftazidime is a bactericidal cephalosporin resistant to most beta-lactanases and active against a wide range of gram positive and gram negative bacteria.

The aim of treatment is to:

1. Identify the infecting organism
2. Apply antibiotics in a concentration that is toxic to the organisms, but not to the retina
3. Prevent further damage to the retina and to the intraocular contents.

The method of treatment will vary depending upon the visual acuity.

### Visual acuity equal to or better than hand movements

In these circumstances, the condition may be treated as follows on an outpatient basis, without recourse to intravenous antibiotics.

1. A vitreous tap is taken through the pars plana for culture and sensitivity
2. Antibiotics are delivered into the vitreal cavity by the same route:
   Amikacin 0.4 mg/0.1 ml saline
   Vancomycin 1.0 mg in 0.1 ml saline

3. The antibiotic onslaught is augmented by subconjunctival injection:
   Vancomycin 25 mg in 0.5 ml saline
   Ceftazidime 100 mg in 0.5 ml saline
4. Vancomycin and amikacin are applied topically
5. Cycloplegics will not only relieve the pain of iris spasm, but will dilate the pupil in case there is a need for intraocular surgery
6. Attempts to limit the damage wrought by infection are based upon corticosteroids:
   Subconjunctival injection of dexamethasone 6 mg in 0.25 ml
   Dexamethasone applied topically
   Systemic prednisolone – 30 mg twice daily for 5–10 days.

If it is not possible to use a vitreous tap with a needle and syringe, then a sample must be collected with the vitreous cutter.

### Visual acuity worse than hand movements

In this case, we move into the realms of pars plana vitrectomy, removing as much of the intravitreal debris as is possible. It must be remembered that the anterior segment may also be involved, and some surgical manipulation may be required to allow a fundal view.

In addition to the vitrectomy the antibiotic/corticosteroid regime described above is instituted.

The majority of cases can be managed without vitrectomy, sometimes on an outpatient basis, and the final outcome will clearly depend to some degree on the type of organism isolated.

### Endogenous metastatic endophthalmitis

The same principles as described for invasional endophthalmitis clearly apply, but the general reduction in the patient's reduced resistance to infection (which led to the condition in the first place) may make successful treatment difficult.

## COMPLICATIONS OF VITRECTOMY

From the moment we decide to carry out vitrectomy, the eye is exposed to several particular dangers.

### Stripping the epithelium of the pars plana

If the in-flow cannula does not enter the cavity of the eye cleanly – a disaster more common when operating on a soft eye – the ciliary epithelium can be stripped from its deep connections. Unless we are aware of the possibility in advance, the first indication might be a huge mound with the scallops of the ora serrata hanging around it like a garland spreading relentlessly across our operating field.

There may be several causes:

1. A sclerotomy through the foothills of the ciliary processes rather than through the pars plana – usually so placed in the hope of preserving the integrity of the ora serrata
2. A short cannula (2.4 mm) uses up much of its length negotiating the sclera and ciliary body, and in a soft eye it may simply be too short to penetrate into the vitreal cavity.

When doubt exists, the following procedures may be of assistance:

1. Injecting air will let us know whether we have penetrated the vitreal cavity
2. Injecting some compatible fluid through the pars plana may raise the pressure of the eye sufficiently to allow the cannula to pass through the ciliary epithelium against resistance.
3. Rotating the cannula and using the angulation of its bevelled tip on entry may help its passage into the correct position.
4. The routine use of a long cannula (4 mm or 6 mm) may clearly penetrate into the vitreal cavity, but its length may cause complications if it is placed too far below the horizontal meridian and damages the lens and the retina.

In an eye that has suffered multiple surgery in the past, it is not always possible to place the cannula correctly, and indeed the decision to enter the vitreal cavity (although wholly justified) may be totally thwarted.

Occasionally the epithelium can be pushed over the sharp end of the cannula by the vitrectomy probe, but such a manoeuvre may create two further complications in place of the single one. The first is traumatic cataract, and the second is a tear in the adjacent retina.

### Aspiration of the retina

If the port hole of the cutter is not continually pointed away from the retina and the retina itself is very mobile, the retina may disappears into the port hole. Not all vitrectomy machines boast a facility to blow the retina back the other way.

### Cataract

A recalcitrant in-flow cannula is not the only danger to the lens. When the vitrectomy probe seeks forwards to remove debris from just behind the lens, it is not surprising that it sometimes goes too far and damages the posterior capsule with the inevitable result.

Prolonged vitrectomy frequently results in cataract in the long term, but some surgical manoeuvres clearly have to be prolonged. It is then a case of balancing the price of an iatrogenic lens opacity against continued vision that would otherwise have been lost.

### Cutting the wrong tissue

To the casual observer, a grey, folded retina can bear an uncanny resemblance to a grey, folded membrane. The presence of retinal vessels can help distinguish the two, and it is better by far to recognize the problem at an early stage than to see (with mounting horror) bare choroid emerging behind what appeared to be successful removal of vitreal debris.

### Bleeding from the entry ports

Care in scleral cautery is of course obligatory, but anticoagulant therapy and bleeding tendencies may further complicate the problem calling for vitrectomy in the first place.

### Hypotony

Whatever the underlying pathology, penetration of the soft eye almost always leads to stripping of the epithelium of the pars plana. Raising the intraocular pressure with intravitreal Ringer's lactate solution or air makes dislodgement of this layer less likely.

## REFERENCES AND FURTHER READING

Charles, S. (1981). *Vitreous Microsurgery*. Williams & Wilkins.

Kasner, D. (1969). Vitrectomy: a new approach to the management of vitreous. *Highlights Ophthalmol.*, **11**, 304.

Machemer, R., Buettner, H., Norton, E. W. D. and Parel, J. M. (1971). Vitrectomy: a pars plana approach. *Tr. Am. Acad. Ophthamol.*, **75**, 813.

Machemer, R., McCuen, B. W. II and de Juan, E. Jnr (1986). Relaxing retinotomies and retinectomies. *Am. J. Ophthalmol.*, **102**, 7.

Rosengren, B. (1966). The silver plomb method in macular hole. *Trans Opth. UK*, **86**, 49.

# 8

# Prophylaxis

It is a medical axiom that prevention is better than cure, but applying this axiom in trying to anticipate a retinal detachment raises problems. Controlled trials concerning ocular disease are ethically difficult, and clinical impressions frequently result in therapeutic rituals that may comfort the doctor but do not necessarily help the patient.

Prophylaxis of retinal disorders might reasonably start with the avoidance of physical injury to all eyes, whether healthy or vulnerable. Thereafter, it consists of interfering with the retina in the hope that the potential danger of doing something is less than the potential danger of doing nothing. Experience tells us that a retina will detach only under a combination of the following conditions:
1. Perforation of the retina
2. Liquifaction and collapse of the vitreous
3. Traction on the retina.

Before we embark on trying to prevent detachment, we must be as sure as possible that conditions do in fact favour it or we may otherwise actually inflict injuries on the eye in the name of treatment.

**Figure 8.1**
A retinal detachment starts in the vitreous, but vitreous collapse does not always lead to a detached retina.

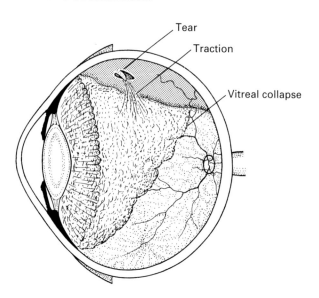

Tear

Traction

Vitreal collapse

In eyes with known lattice degeneration, it is remarkable how the retina may remain flat for years and then tear in a totally unexpected place. If this occurs following prophylactic interference, then the hardest part of the surgery is explaining to the patient how it happened. Indeed, if there has been an unhappy surgical result in the first eye it is clinically wiser not to interfere with the fellow eye, but to wait for things to develop in the full expectation that they will do so.

Should we decide on prophylactic intervention, we must then consider the courses of action that are available to us. The inflammatory reaction is best provided by cryopexy (as in a fullblown detachment), but may equally be provided by laser if the media are clear enough and the patient sufficiently tolerant.


## CRYOPEXY

This is usually a non-sterile procedure, carried out via the conjunctiva. Generalized sedation is required only for the extremely nervous, and the only anaesthesia necessary after topical application is local subconjunctival infiltration.

The conjunctival sac will, of course, prevent cryopexy behind the equator. If for some reason (e.g. hazy media) light cannot be used, then the conjunctiva must be opened. At this point the procedure becomes a sterile one, but it is reasonable to try more extensive local infiltration of anaesthetic before proceeding to retrobulbar injection.

**Fig 8.2**
Posterior seeking by the cryoprobe is limited by the conjunctival fornix. If the tear is too posterior to reach, the conjunctiva must be opened at the limbus under aseptic conditions to permit access.

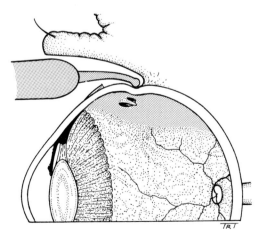


## LASER PHOTOCOAGULATION

Unless delivered using the indirect ophthalmoscope, laser coagulation must be carried out with the help of either a three-mirror or pan-fundoscopic contact lens. It goes without saying that this technique can only be performed if the retina is flat, and there is little to choose between the two techniques from the point of view of adhesive strength.

## ENCIRCLING BAND

If traction is deemed the major danger, an encircling silicone band might be the more sensible form of intervention. This is because coagulation alone is not wholly benign, and may indeed shrink the vitreous cortex, resulting in traction or (worse still) the very detachment it seeks to prevent.

To state the obvious, the great dilemma is to know what to treat, how to treat it, whether to treat it, and if so, when to do so?

## APPEARANCES NOT REQUIRING TREATMENT

### Microcystoid degeneration
This is found in all eyes. It lies at the extreme retinal periphery, and its name makes no other description necessary. It is benign, and only rarely spreads to form larger, smooth-walled cysts in the outer plexiform layer of the retina – also benign.

### Chorioretinal degeneration
This name applies to the 'black pepper' pigment that lies behind the microcysts, or which may cover the retinal periphery by itself.

**Figure 8.3**
Pigment stippling in the peripheral retina is normal, and is routinely picked up with the binocular indirect ophthalmoscope.

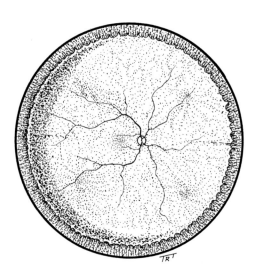

**Figure 8.4**
Benign equatorial pigmentary
degeneration is common, and has no
serious significance.

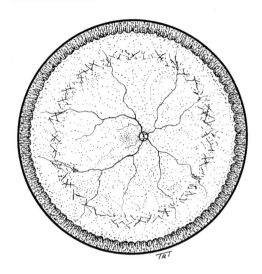

### Benign equatorial pigmentary degeneration
In older age groups, a fine-spun interlacing pattern of mottled pigmentation encircles the globe around the equator. This might be seen with the direct ophthalmoscope through the dilated pupil, and the danger is that casual observation may lead to a mistaken diagnosis of retinitis pigmentosa.

The pigmentary scatter of this degeneration implies self-induced adhesions of the retina to the choroid.

### Paving stone degeneration
These disc-like white patches are found on the peripheral retina in middle age. Although atrophic the ocular layers stick together, despite giving the constant impression of imminent perforation.

### White with pressure
The name indicates the colour and occurrence of this condition. It is commonly found surrounding the posterior border of microcystoid degeneration, when the scleral depressor is at work. Isolated oblong patches may appear when the mound produced by the depressor reaches the equator. There are differing opinions on its significance, but it probably indicates that the retina is not healthy in these areas. It therefore merits careful watching, lest definite evidence of vitreoretinal adhesions (such as flashing lights) shows it to be the forerunner of a retinal tear. The nearer the patch to the equator, the greater the likelihood of this eventuality.

The slope of the examining mound towards the disc may show up as white in a heavily pigmented fundus. In this case, the retina is merely showing its translucent profile against the dark background.

**Figure 8.5**
Paving stone degeneration.The
underlying process which causes
atrophy of the ocular layers happily
results in their adhesion to each
other.

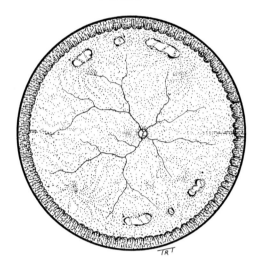

**Figure 8.6**
The significance of white with or
without pressure is still a matter of
controversy. If it appears in an area of
previous detachment it must be
regarded as a suggestion, if not a
sign, of possible leakage of fluid into
the subretinal space.

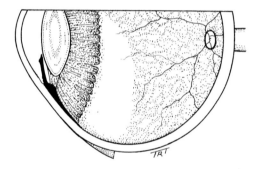

### White without pressure

As might be guessed from the name, the appearance can be
seen using the indirect ophthalmoscope, without the need for
scleral depression. In most cases it is probably benign, but
occasionally it is the first evidence of subretinal fluid seeping
downwards from a tiny retinal break. Any progression must
be regarded as the start of a detachment, taking it out of this
section and into the group of appearances that may require
treatment.

### Retinoschisis and retinal cysts

There are few conditions as mystifying as the cystic retina –
both in knowing what to call it, and what to do about it.

### Senile retinoschisis

Senile retinoschisis results from a split in the outer plexiform
layer of the retina, and gives rise to bilateral, smooth, often
enormous balloon elevations, commonly – but by no means
always – found in the lower temporal quadrants. White dots

**Figure 8.7**
A retinoschisis is smooth-walled, a detachment ripples, and a combination of the two is sometimes possible. Treatment of any retinal detachment is directed to the outer leaf break.

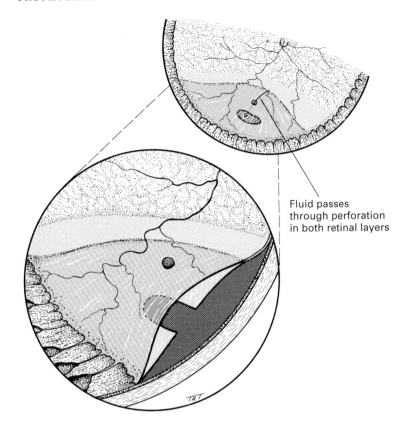

Fluid passes through perforation in both retinal layers

scattered throughout the domes of these elevations are called 'snowflakes', and are thought to represent the remnants of the cells that once bound the layers together.

The condition is asymptomatic, and almost always benign. However, if breaks develop in both layers of the retina, a frank detachment adds a rippling elevation to the smooth elevation. The appearance then becomes one of a shallow detachment in the outer leaf, producing a creamy grey rippling reflex in which a large rounded tear is often visible, the whole complex faintly obscured by the snowflake cyst lying over it in the vitreal cavity. Any treatment must be directed to the outer leaf break.

Cryopexy picks up the outer leaf in a very characteristic dimpled polka-dot pattern. The white background is studded with dark circles as regularly distributed as the holes in a colander.

### Juvenile retinoschisis

This is a hereditary condition, and is included in this section for convenience and because, like senile retinoschisis, it does not call for prophylaxis. What it does need is actual treatment, which may not be very effective. The split occurs in the inner plexiform layer, and its progression is as destructive of peripheral vision as is the coexistent macular degeneration of the central area.

### Retinal cysts

These are marked by their rarity, occurring (if at all) as concomitants of long-standing retinal detachments, forming between the whole thickness retina and a layer of connective tissue. Their edges are round and sharp, unlike the blurred margin of a true detachment, and in themselves they require no treatment. If the underlying detachment is treatable, it should be treated and the cyst will then take care of itself.

## APPEARANCES WHICH MAY REQUIRE TREATMENT

Abnormal adhesions between the vitreous and the retina, usually around the equator, produce the multiple appearances of lattice degeneration. The classic name comes from the white crisscross line patterns that make the appearance unforgettable, but the fanciful notion of a gastropod trailing across the equator and leaving a snail track behind it is just as common. If the lattice is significant, it may produce tears in two ways.

Round holes are the result of simple asymptomatic atrophy. They may stop at this point, or may slowly progress, giving the retina time to circle them with round 'tide marks'. These may well break clear, giving rise to a frank retinal detachment, or (more commonly still) they may remain asymptomatic until a chance discovery raises the dilemma of what to do about them.

**Figure 8.8**
Lattice degeneration, in all its manifestations, is not in itself an indication for treatment.

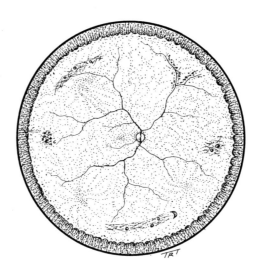

Horseshoe breaks follow traction forces, which pull the lattice towards the vitreal cavity. The traction causes flashing lights, and if a break follows it tends to be symptomatic, if not dramatic, with floaters due to haemorrhage or retinal pigment, and/or a frank retinal detachment.

However, it is well known (even more so since Byers' protracted and meticulous survey) that most lattice change gives rise more to anxiety than it does to retinal breaks. Should a detachment ever occur in an eye with lattice degeneration, the chances are that some remote and unsuspected area of retina is to blame.

### Retinal breaks

These of course are *the sine qua non* of a rhegmatogenous retinal detachment, but all breaks do not lead to retinal detachment, being present in 7–8% of trouble-free eyes.

Horseshoe tears are more likely to give rise to retinal elevation, because their shape implies vitreoretinal traction. Round holes are less dangerous, and certainly less symptomatic.

## WHEN AND WHEN NOT TO INTERFERE

When breaks and retinal degeneration are associated with retinal separation, management has gone beyond the stage of prophylaxis and there is now only one possible decision.

When no separation of the retina exists, then the choices of action multiply. It is clear that operating and claiming successful intervention when nothing would have happened anyway is as much an error of judgement as sparking off preretinal retraction in an otherwise asymptomatic eye.

It is probably wise to use prophylaxis sparingly and only then for reasons convincing to both doctor and patient.

When one retina has already come adrift, intervention is indicated in the fellow eye in two sets of circumstances:
1. If the fellow retina also has a break
2. If the fellow eye has a potential tear in a mirror image position to that causing the first detachment.

A 'potential tear' is described as:
1. An area of lattice change
2. Retinal distortion that might be construed as a tear in the making
3. The retinal periphery of an eye, the fellow of which has suffered a giant tear.

When neither retina has detached, prophylaxis should be considered for the following:
1. All symptomatic horseshoe breaks
2. Upper temporal breaks which might threaten the macula

3. When there is widespread lattice change (particularly with multiple round holes) encircling the retina along the equatorial contour line.

The resolve to treat is strengthened in the following cases:
1. Myopia
2. Vitreous degeneration and collapse
3. A family tendency to retinal separation.

Vitreal degeneration is by far the most important of these three conditions.

Interference depends on what is perceived as the greater danger – the languid seepage of fluid into the subretinal space, or actual retinal traction. If it is the former, then simple co-agulation may be considered reasonable. If it is the latter, then an encircling silicone band – either on its own or accompanied by judicious coagulation – may be thought the wiser course.

For all other appearances, benign neglect is probably better for most patients than routine interference in the name of treatment.

## REFERENCES AND FURTHER READING

Byer, N. E. (1982). The natural history of asymptomatic retinal breaks. *Ophthalmology*, **89**, 1033–1039.

Chignell, A. H. and Shilling, J. S. (1973). Prophylaxis of retinal detachment. *Br. J. Ophthalmol.*, **57**, 291–298.

Morse, P. H. and Scheie, H. G. (1974). Prophylactic cryoretinopathy of retinal breaks. *Arch. Ophthalmol.*, **92**, 204–207.

# 9

# Hazards – how to recover

THICKENED POSTERIOR CAPSULE

Any retina viewed through a thickened posterior capsule tends to appear detached.

*Management*
1. Avoid Yag capsulotomy in principle unless the vision is seriously hampered.
2. Confirm absence of detachment by the following:
   (a) Normal hand movement field
   (b) Absence of slit lamp signs in the anterior chamber or anterior vitreous
   (c) Equal intraocular pressures
   (d) B Scan ultrasound, if fundal examination is completely uninformative.

VITREAL HAEMORRHAGE

In the absence of diabetes, hypertension or any of the bleeding disorders, we must assume the cause to be either a retinal break alone or a retinal break with detachment.

*Management*
Blood lingering in the vitreal cavity may well be the trigger to subsequent proliferative vitreoretinopathy. There are two options to prevent this:
1. Early vitrectomy will identify and deal with the cause quickly, and is generally the favoured choice.
2. More conservatively, B scan ultrasound, if indicating a flat retina, may be repeated at regular intervals (if the patient can tolerate the delay) until a clearing haemorrhage indicates what has happened.

## REOPERATION

The best chance of a successful operation is the first chance. The main difficulty with second or third chance surgery is that of access.

*Management*
1. Adhesions behind the limbus make it necessary to open the conjunctiva further back than is either usual or desirable. After surgery, single stitch conjunctival closure may not adequately cover any scleral explants. When late exposure of such explants is anticipated, it is best to bring the anterior and posterior conjunctival edges into apposition and hold them there with as many vicryl (polybutylate) sutures as necessary.
2. Scleral dissection, when strictly necessary, limits post-operative morbidity.
3. Multiple surgery of the scleral surface obscures anatomical detail in an all-embracing membrane. Nibbling through this membrane with blunt-tipped scissors will again reveal the natural cleavage line between the rectus muscles and the sclera, and the muscle edge can then be picked up in a St. Martin's forceps.
4. The entire width of each rectus muscle must be identified lest it be split by a stay suture.
5. Adhesions deep to the muscle insertion must be cleared before insertion of a squint hook is attempted. The sclera in this area is particularly fragile.
6. It is critical never to lose control of the needle tip of the stay suture, or it may perforate the retina.

   **NB:** The superior oblique muscle (almost always anterior to its normal position) never fails to be caught on a squint hook – particularly one approaching from the nasal side.

## RAISED INTRAOCULAR PRESSURE – BEFORE SURGERY

In most cases retinal detachment reduces the intraocular pressure, but if there is unsuspected raised pressure, it can lead to incarceration of the retina during subretinal fluid release.

*Management*
A raised intraocular pressure must be reduced before surgery with one of the following:
1. Topical anti-glaucoma drugs
2. Systemic acetazolamide
3. Mannitol (rarely used).

## POOR FUNDAL VIEW

### Corneal haze
Apart from pre-existing corneal disease, there are two main causes of corneal haze:
1. Eyelids left open between the induction of anaesthesia and surgery
2. Damage to the epithelium, which is particularly vulnerable in diabetics, during the opening manoeuvres of peritomy and threading of the stay sutures.

*Management*
Surgery may still be possible although the view is obscured, but removal of the epithelium will make the operation both more likely to succeed and quicker – it must be completed within the 45 minutes remaining before the view is obscured for a second and final time.

### Intraoperative raised intraocular pressure
Intraocular pressure which rises during surgery results in a waterlogged cornea. Such oedema, occurring in vulnerable eyes, is also aggravated by the following:
1. Cryopexy (which may also close the central retinal artery), during each application
2. The injection of air into the vitreous
3. The application of a scleral buckle in the absence of sufficient space.

*Management*
1. Paracentesis.
2. Reduction of the intravitreal bubble.
3. Slackening of the tension sutures.

### Cataract
The lens opacity, whilst allowing the identification of a retinal detachment, may prevent its treatment.

*Management*
Cataract extraction with or without a lens implant is inescapable. Even a small incision technique will require temporary strengthening of the corneoscleral suture if the wound is to survive the retinal operation.

### Frog spawn bubbles in the anterior chamber
In aphakic eyes or where the iris lens diaphragm is imperfect, multiple bubbles can bring surgery to a halt by obscuring the view.

*Management*
1. Anticipate the problem, and verify and remember the important landmarks that will vanish behind these infuriating little beads.
2. Although it is an additional procedure, temporary replacement of the air with a balanced salt solution may allow the frustrated operation to be resumed.

NB: A single movement of the plunger in a dry syringe, using a dry needle, will usually produce a single bubble.

### Pupil will not dilate
Such pupils are adequate for seeing out but hopeless for seeing in, and are not infrequently found in the following circumstances:
1. Eyes of diabetics
2. Eyes which have suffered previous anterior chamber inflammation
3. Eyes subjected to long-term treatment with pilocarpine.

*Management*
1. Phenylephrine (2.5–10%, if permitted by the anaesthetist) should be dropped onto the sclera. It should not be dropped on the cornea, where its effect on the epithelium will reduce the view still further.
2. If mydriatics fail, then a sector iridectomy should permit adequate visualization of the fundus – provided there is no attendant anterior chamber haemorrhage.
3. Iris microhooks introduced through corneal stab incisions in the four quadrants can mechanically produce a view that cannot be achieved with mydriatics.

### Anterior chamber haemorrhage due to paracentesis
An entry point near the limbus may allow limbal vessels to discharge blood into the anterior chamber.

*Management*
A balanced salt solution, passed through an anterior chamber maintainer and through the lower cornea into the anterior chamber, will clear the blood very efficiently. **NB:** It may also touch the lens.

## BREAKS NOT FOUND

Despite searching in the correct places, a retinal break is not always discovered.

*Management*
Softening the eye by paracentesis makes indentation easier, and also frequently makes it easier to locate breaks that would otherwise remain concealed. The search can also be made easier psychologically for the surgeon if carried out in a considered fashion. Those areas where breaks are not expected should be examined quickly and dismissed first, leaving the mind free to concentrate on the more likely areas.

## BREAKS STILL NOT FOUND

When the most diligent of searches still reveals nothing, we must ensure that there is no underlying tumour or exudation.

*Management*
There is no single approach, but it is reasonable to apply cryopexy to those areas where breaks are predicted by the Gonin–Lincoff–Gieser rules. Thereafter, the following procedures may be carried out if appropriate:
1. Subretinal fluid release – which might incidentally unmask a coy break.
2. Use of intravitreal air/gas.
3. Application of a scleral buckle.

## RAISED INTRAOCULAR PRESSURE DURING SURGERY

Pressure from the cryoprobe raises the pressure within the eye sufficiently to close the central retinal artery during each application. Such traction must be released before the vital moment when the choroidal knuckle is perforated, otherwise the subretinal fluid will sweep the retina into the channel intended for its own passage.

Scleral buckling after an injection of air may call for more space than is available. The eye may become taut like a drum, and in these circumstances it is dangerously easy to pass a needle intended for the sclera through the retina.

*Management*
1. Anticipation of the problem.
2. Removal of some intravitreal air.
3. Paracentesis.

## NEEDLE THROUGH THE CHOROID/ CHORIORETINA

The most carefully placed scleral needle can sometimes pass to the deep surface of a thin sclera – a problem made more likely by attempting to suture an eye that is either too soft or too hard.

There are three essential dangers:
1. The actual perforation of the retina
2. A haemorrhage tracking down to the macula
3. The possible association between tractional detachment and intravitreal bleeding.

Maddeningly, the very steps taken to try to ensure safety can sometimes lead directly to a different danger. For example, if a detachment is too shallow for the safe release of subretinal fluid, a paracentesis (to make space) or air into the vitreous (to seal the tear) might be considered. This averts one danger, but there is now the risk of applying scleral sutures to a hard eye.

The sensation of a needle passing onto the wrong surface of the sclera is unmistakable, and requires no description – nor indeed does the sight of fluid flowing unplanned from the same needle track.

### Management
Haemorrhage (although not inevitable) must be assumed and immediately contained, and the following steps carried out:
1. Increase the air to the vitreal cavity to raise the intraocular pressure.
2. Identify the damage.
3. Apply cryopexy to the new retinal perforation.
4. Place the scleral buckle to catch the new perforation, remembering that a paracentesis to reduce the intraocular pressure must come before the application of a new scleral suture.

## RETINAL DETACHMENT WITH UPPER HORSESHOE BREAK

### Management
1. Bed rest, to protect the macula and help predict subsequent retinal behaviour.
2. Cryopexy.
3. Subretinal fluid release (optional).
4. Intravitreal air (optional).
5. Scleral buckle (space made with paracentesis, fluid release as the eye dictates).

6. Check the same contour line for secondary breaks.
7. Multiple breaks are best caught on the anterior slope of an encircling band.

## RETINAL DETACHMENT WITH LOWER HORSESHOE BREAK

Whilst gravity before surgery protects the macula, after surgery it may encourage the collection of subretinal fluid around the still-open break. For this reason, scleral buckling without fluid release may be unsuccessful. It is always best to see the break stretched dry across the indentation at the end of the operation.

It should also be remembered that an air bubble will not float downwards. A large bubble, however, may achieve some degree of flotation with the patient lying on one side or the other, and with the foot of the bed elevated.

### Management

As for upper horseshoe breaks, with the proviso that stretching the break dry will usually call for subretinal fluid release.

## MULTIPLE BREAKS

Breaks in all quadrants, on different contour lines, and usually in high myopes, spell trouble. Simple conventional surgery, which may well succeed in flattening the retina for a while, is usually followed by recurrence of the detachment about six weeks later.

### Management

1. Warn the patient in advance, with guarded optimism.
2. Vitrectomy – to make space, relieve traction and remove surface membranes.
3. Laser photocoagulation if the retina can be flattened, or cryocoagulation if it cannot.
4. A broad, encircling buckle – a guttered explant (287 in the Mira catalogue) – or a half-thickness 7 mm silastic sponge, joined with a clove hitch. The aim of both of these, the latter being higher and broader, is to catch all the breaks on the indent.

### The six-weeks' recurrence

If the retina detaches again despite the measures described above, then the major causal element has to be traction.

## Management
1. If the breaks can be closed with an even higher buckle, then silicone oil should not pass through them to the deep surface of the retina.
2. If the breaks cannot be closed, then heavy liquid (in a bubble) expanding over the optic nerve head will flatten the retina.
3. Encircling laser photocoagulation may hold the retina in position after removal of the heavy liquid.
4. If such a hope is unlikely to be realized, then silicone oil may be substituted – permanently – for the heavy liquid.

## SUBRETINAL FLUID TOO DEEP

In this situation, cryopexy cannot be accurately applied.

## Management
1. Check the scleral landmarks of intravitreal positions in case the fundal view is subsequently obscured.
2. Release subretinal fluid, to make the detachment more shallow.
3. Insert intravitreal air, to:
   (a) restore the ocular volume
   (b) seal the breaks later.
4. When the detachment is shallow enough, apply cryopexy.
5. Add whatever buckling might be deemed appropriate.

## SUBRETINAL FLUID TOO SHALLOW

## Management
1. Paracentesis, to make space.
2. Vitrectomy.

The twin dangers here relate to the release of subretinal fluid, and the absence of space for necessary retinal manoeuvres. Attempting fluid release can lead to incarceration of the retina, resulting in a new hole in the retina which has only one saving grace in that its exact position is known.

### Incarceration leading to perforation of the retina
## Management
1. Cryopexy to the iatrogenic retinal perforation.
2. Scleral imbrication or the addition of a scleral buckle, if considered safer.
3. Intravitreal air. This may well have been injected for the primary detachment and therefore performs two duties.

## DRY TAP

Subretinal fluid, which is always happily released in text-books, may not necessarily appear to order in the operating room.

*Management*
If no subretinal fluid flows, then the sclerotomy must be sutured and abandoned. The surgeon must under no circumstances probe into the vitreal cavity, hoping of turning a dry tap into a wet one.

## FAILED CLOSURE OF BREAK WITHOUT SUBRETINAL FLUID RELEASE

**During surgery**
This occurs when the retinal break continues to stand proud of the buckle.

*Management*
Make space, using one of the following methods:
1. Paracentesis.
2. Subretinal fluid release, if the fluid is very deep or the break is in the lower quadrants.
3. Intravitreal air, if the break is in the upper quadrants.

**After surgery**
In this case, there are two likely causes: either the retina is not mobile (poor surgical judgement), or the buckle is in the wrong place.

*Management*
1. Give the retina 24 hours grace to settle.
2. If it does not, return to the operating theatre for the following:
    (a) subretinal fluid release (if the intraocular pressure is safe)
    (b) to check that the buckle is accurately placed.
    (c) to add intravitreal air (if space be available).

## MAKING SPACE

Conventional manoeuvres may fail if the subretinal fluid is too shallow, or if the retinal procedures demand more space than is available.

*Management*
1. Paracentesis will probably be inadequate.
2. Subretinal fluid release is not possible in these circumstances.
3. Vitrectomy is always safer than the attempted release of subretinal fluid where not enough fluid exists.

## HYPOTONY

In the abscence of a frank scleral rupture, an eye may be soft due to ciliary shock. Such an eye may not tolerate vigorous manipulation.

Two further difficulties present themselves. Attempting to place a suture in the sclera will throw the ocular layers into folds, which may allow the needle to perforate all the layers – including the retina. Also, placing a vitrectomy inflow can strip the epithelium of the pars plana.

*Management*
A sharp needle can sometimes pass safely without separating the ciliary epithelium, and air or Ringer's lactate may be injected through this to raise the intraocular pressure sufficiently for necessary manoeuvres to be carried out. Indeed, raising the pressure of such an eye may well be beneficial and boost the ciliary body into renewed function.

If vitrectomy is decided upon, a 6 mm inflow may certainly avoid stripping the epithelium, but only at the expense of threatening the lens and the retina instead. Both of these will survive intact if the inflow is not angled needlessly in either direction.

## HARD EYE

Scleral buckling and air injection may sometimes 'overfill' the eye. Apart from the threat to the central retinal artery, a taut sclera will not allow the needle tip dimpling necessary to gauge scleral depth. If the raised pressure is due to intravitreal air, the sclera takes on a drum-like quality, and is almost resonant.

*Management*
1. Paracentesis.
2. Reduce the intravitreal bubble.
3. Slacken the tension sutures.

## SUPRACHOROIDAL COLLECTIONS

These may be collections of air, infusion fluid or blood.

### Air
The air injection needle must pass cleanly into the vitreal cavity, otherwise it may strip the ciliary epithelium – and possibly the retina – resulting in a subretinal air bubble, or separate the entire ciliary body from the sclera, resulting in a suprachoroidal air bubble.

The subretinal air is recognized as a transparent bubble rolling beneath the neuroretina. Full-thickness choroidal detachments, whatever the cause, look very similar to one other.

#### *Management*
1. Recognize the problem.
2. If sufficient space remains to complete the operation, the ectopic air may be ignored.
3. If yet more space is required, then the subretinal air has to be released in the same way as subretinal fluid.

### Infusion line choroidal detachment
The Ringer's lactate accumulates in the suprachoroidal space, where it should not, thereby raising a mound in the vitreal cavity.

#### *Management*
1. Recognize the problem.
2. Position a longer inflow at a different site, if possible.

### Suprachoroidal haemorrhage
The causes are many, including:
1. Hypertension, whether unsuspected or established
2. Anticoagulant therapy
3. Excessive cryopexy
4. Hypotony.

Extreme bleeding may track forwards into the anterior chamber, raising the intraocular pressure and threatening to stain the cornea unless contained urgently.

#### *Management*
1. Anticipation.
2. The common run of topical antiglaucoma drops will have no effect, although pilocarpine might well open the drainage angle – at the expense of obscuring the retinal view.
3. Latanoprost, a synthetic prostaglandin, might possibly bypass the blocked trabecular meshwork by selectively increasing uveoscleral outflow.

4. If the intraocular pressure cannot be reduced, the anterior chamber blood must be washed out with a balanced salt solution through an anterior chamber maintainer. Be aware that such a manoeuvre risks causing a cataract.

Cataract extraction and lens implantation are best done at this stage, if they appear inescapable, rather than at another operation. The blood in the suprachoroidal space may then be drained if possible by sclerotomy over the pars plans.

The presence of vitreal blood requires vitrectomy to allow the accurate location of choroidal detachments. However, this presupposes the possibility of setting up an infusion line, which may well prove impossible.

## APHAKIC BREAK(S)

Extracapsular extraction complicated by vitreous loss or by subsequent Yag capsulotomy may result in small tears at the root of the vitreous base. These tears are recognized as little wisps like goats' beards on the summit of the scleral depressor behind the ora serrata.

### Management
Encirclement is always the best option for such eyes.

## THIN SCLERA

Common in myopes, the thin sclera is almost always found where it matters – directly over the retinal break.

### Management
It is in these circumstances that an encircling band comes into its own, because the tension sutures required to indent with a guttered explant can, by using the rectus insertions, at least avoid suspect sclera anterior to the buckle. Placing the band with much safer holding sutures can in turn put the buckle where it is required.

## CRYOPEXY FAILING TO PRODUCE AN END POINT

Although the fault may be in the cryo machine itself, it is far more likely to lie with surgical failure to clear the scleral surface. More effective cryopexy can be achieved by pressing the probe firmly onto the globe at the beginning of the cycle of freezing, thus eliminating any water between the probe and the sclera.

It must be remembered that the pressure closes the central retinal artery each time cryopexy is applied, and this pressure must be relaxed the moment the freeze has started.

Precision with the cryoprobe is similar to that achieved by an expert putter. If the direction of the forefinger corresponds directly to that of the cryoprobe tip, then there should be never any doubt as to where that tip is pointing. This will allow many episodes of a single application, as desired, rather than a few unwanted applications.

## KISSING CHOROIDAL DETACHMENTS

Compression of the vortex by tight encirclement may lead to mutual contact of the retina, draped over broad choroidal mounds, in the mid vitreal cavity of the retina. A painful eye suggests associated anterior segment ischaemia.

### Management
1. Inactivity, if the mounds do not actually touch and are seen to be receding.
2. If the mounds continue to advance, the band must be slackened, or – if it is easier – cut, particularly if ischaemia seems possible.

## FISH MOUTHING OF A RETINAL BREAK

Such redundant folding of the retina used to be regarded as one of the major complications of circumferential explants. The cause lies in the reduction of the ocular circumference, without any corresponding reduction in the retinal area. This condition is perhaps most commonly found when the centre point of a dialysis or disinsertion, peaks like a gothic arch above the indentation.

### Management
1. Injection of air into the vitreous and subsequent head down positioning almost always closes the break.
2. If it appears that it will not, then the addition of a fragment of silastic sponge deep to the scleral explant may augment closure from the outside.

## CENTRAL ARTERY OCCLUSION

This occurs during surgery on eyes where the arterial circulation is compromised (as in chronic glaucoma), or where there is not enough space for the necessary retinal manoeuvres. Recurrent fundal examination to monitor the effect of manoeuvres is a familiar feature of retinal surgery, but checking the patency of the central retinal artery must take precedence over them all. Critical signs are pulsing of the artery, which (with increasing pressure) gives way to blanching of the optic nerve head. Such evidence of ischaemia is ignored at the patient's peril.

### Management
A closed artery is a matter of urgency, and the following procedures must be performed at once.
1. Paracentesis.
2. Some intravitreal air, if present, should be removed through the pars plana via the same syringe and needle with which it was injected.
3. Should neither of the above prove sufficient, then release of the buckling sutures will open the arterial flow once more.

## CONTINUED LOSS OF FLUID VITREOUS

If little formed vitreous remains in an eye, sclerotomy for subretinal fluid release directly over a break will occasionally result in the passage of fluid from the vitreal cavity. If this is not contained, it could empty the eye to the point of collapse.

### Management
1. Anticipate the problem, if a fluid flow continues longer than might have been expected.
2. Inject air into the vitreous whilst the eye is still firm enough to allow the safe passage of a needle through the pars plana.
3. Stitch the sclerotomy.
4. Turn the unexpectedly large space achieved to the benefit of the eye by using more air than originally intended.
5. Complete the buckling, removing the sclerotomy stitch from below the explant at the last moment. Suture material left deep to a buckle may appear inertly and benignly in the vitreal cavity as the years pass.

## RAISED INTRAOCULAR PRESSURE AFTER SURGERY

This may have several causes:
1. Heavy encirclement may block the flow from the vortex ampullae into the vortex veins
2. Forward movement of the iris lens diaphragm in a vulnerable eye can block the drainage angle.
3. Blood in the anterior chamber can silt up the trabecular meshwork.

### Management
1. Topical antiglaucoma medications may control the pressure until the ocular fluid flow comes into balance.
2. If these drugs fail, then the buckle may have to be slackened (and the retina may redetach).
3. Red blood cells in the anterior chamber (not in the presence of raised pressure) threaten the corneal clarity, and may by their continued presence keep the pressure elevated. In these circumstances, an anterior chamber washout with a balanced salt solution through an anterior chamber maintainer will restore the view.

## GENERAL PRINCIPLES

Should new circumstances develop by chance, it is a surgical refinement to turn these to the benefit of the eye in question, if possible. For example, inadvertent subretinal fluid release, whilst not a planned part of the procedure, may of course result from a new hole in the retina. It also, however, produces extra space that was not anticipated, and this space should be gratefully accepted and used in the continuing procedure.

It must be remembered that – apart from operating on a doctor, a nurse or the spouse of either! – the commonest cause of complications is the complacent assumption that they will not happen. Remember, a simple retinal detachment is one that is not yet complicated.

# Epilogue

The cornerstone of retinal detachment surgery is to know where the causal breaks can be found, and how to see them in relation to all the contents of the vitreal cavity. Seeing the distribution, the contours, hollows and quality of a detached retina is the first step to understanding what to do about it. This includes understanding that there is no such thing as a single operation, but rather a series of legitimate manoeuvres that may be used alone, in sequence or in combination, depending upon the eye in question.

The manoeuvres are not complicated, despite an abiding conviction that they ought to be. The secret, if there be one, is to recognize that each stratagem can have a secondary influence which may be used to our advantage. For example, air in the vitreous can seal a tear by surface tension. It can also make up the intraocular volume either at leisure or in a hurry, and to the observant surgeon its rate of absorption can give matchless information about the intraocular pressure.

Once the reason why takes precedence over ritual, the surgery of retinal detachment becomes a pleasure – not just in flourishing a technical skill, but in sharing the delight of those whose sight has been preserved because of it.

# Index